NO EXCUSES!
50 Healthy Ways to
ROCK Breakfast!

50 simple recipes
to get lean and healthy

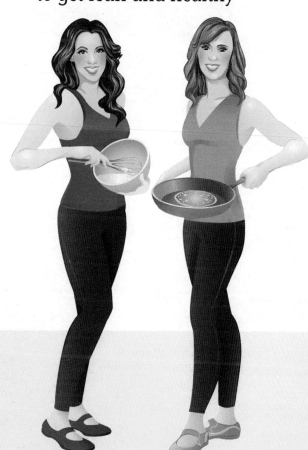

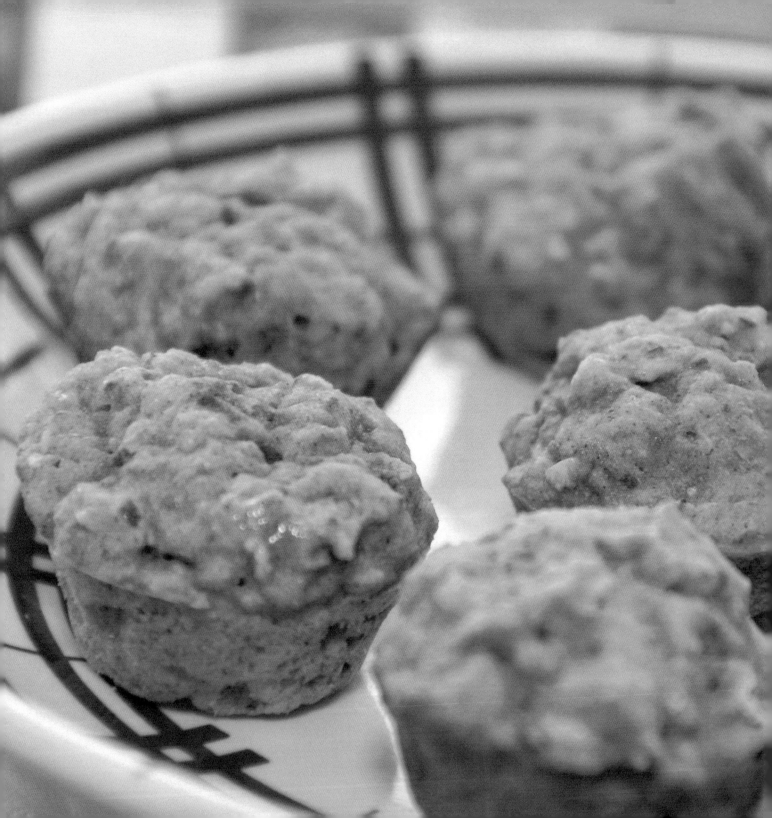

NO EXCUSES!

50 Healthy Ways to ROCK Breakfast!

50 Breakfast Recipes
that will change your body for good!!

The U ROCK GIRLS share their secrets
to healthy living

The easy way to ROCK a healthy body
is to start your day in a healthy way

"One of the biggest obstacles people face when trying to eat healthy is the amount of time and investment of energy it takes. Tiffani and Erin call your bluff in this new book by making the first meal of the day extremely easy and simple. Now you have no excuse not to rock breakfast with advice and insight from these two RDs who I've had a pleasure working with over the past few years."

~**James Patrick,** ACS, ALB AAFT Gold Addy®
 Award Winning Photographer

"Before, I viewed cooking as a chore and found it difficult to prepare a meal that was both healthy and satisfying at the same time. Erin and Tiffani have taught me you do not need to skimp on flavor to be healthy. By selecting fresh produce, herbs and cooking with a variety of ingredients to pull out a food's natural flavors, one really doesn't have to sacrifice flavor. Erin and Tiffani are cooking up more than great food….They are cooking up an awareness that eating healthy and achieving wellness is truly within grasp."

~**Christine Trautmann,** Cooking class devotee, wife, mom,
and U Rock Girl subscriber

"Erin and Tiff are two of the shining stars of healthy eating! Their creativity jumps out of the pages of their book. I have relied on them for years for nutrition education, collaboration and inspiration."

~**Cathy Savage,** International Fitness Coach and Entrepreneur

Table of Contents

Acknowledgements

There are so many people we want to thank for supporting us in pouring our time and passion into this book. Without their patience, understanding and expertise, this book could not have gone from our heart to paper.

THANK YOU TO:

Our families:

Erin's family: Fabulous hubby **Scott;** awesome foursome of boys **Eric, Ryan, Alex, Jax.**

Tiffani's family: Super-husband **Dan;** kiddo three-pack **Dylan, Emily, Riley.**

Erin's sister (and *Tiff's cousin*) **Kelli Schatz** for her "real woman" perspective.

Alison Plotnik for shooting the beautiful photographs in the Arizona heat!

Food stylists **Diana Draper** and **Erin Becker** for turning your artistic vision into mouth watering photographs.

Rachel Hoffer for allowing us to invade her beautiful kitchen.

Creative editor and good friend, **Diane Watson,** for her insight and experience.

......o......

Joe Bardin, our editor, for guiding us through this adventure.

......o......

Claudia Gimenez, our graphic designer, whose generosity with her talents gave life to our ideas.

......o......

Our parents, **Denise** and **Ernie, Suzi** and **Pops, Jimmy** and **Sally,** for raising us, loving us, supporting us, and putting us through school so we could become Registered Dietitian Nutritionists!

......o......

Our grandparents, **Nany Sony** and **Papa Ben,** for inspiring this book. Your love, time, and countless sleepovers, cultivated our love and passion for breakfast. **Nany,** you were the original dietitian in the family (as you told us many times)!

......o......

Casey O'Neill, Ashley Patterson, and **Amanda Vaughn,** our interns who tirelessly researched, analyzed and toiled endlessly.

......o......

Foreword

I'm a huge fan of breakfast. In fact--and I know I'm not the first person in the fitness industry to admit this--sometimes just the thought of hot oatmeal or fluffy scrambled eggs when I wake up in the morning is incentive for me to go to sleep. Which is why I couldn't be more excited for the release of this cookbook. It not only drives home the importance of starting the day with a solid meal, but it also offers up 50 healthy and satisfying ways to do so. But what makes this book so special are the strong and talented women behind it. In the last few years, Tiffani and Erin have become my go-to experts for professional dietary advice and incredible recipes that help women fuel their active lifestyles and maintain a healthy body. I can always rely on them to take a delicious idea and put a creative spin on it to ensure that the dish is packed with nutrients without compromising the pleasure and joy of eating. Many of their recipes that I've published have become reader favorites, and repeats in my own meal plans. It's clear in the quality of their work, these two inspiring women love what they do. They are shining examples that a healthy, beautiful life doesn't require crash dieting or eliminating your favorite foods. Instead, it's not about what you take out of your diet, but what you put into it: a variety of colorful, whole foods, that benefit your body so you can perform optimally in everything you do. And it all starts with a good breakfast.

As a former nutrition editor for Oxygen Magazine, I could always count on Tiffani and Erin to provide nutritious and delicious recipes for our readers in their Easy Does It column. Here are samples of a few of my favorite articles.

Kirstyn Brown
Editor-in-Chief
STRONG Fitness Magazine

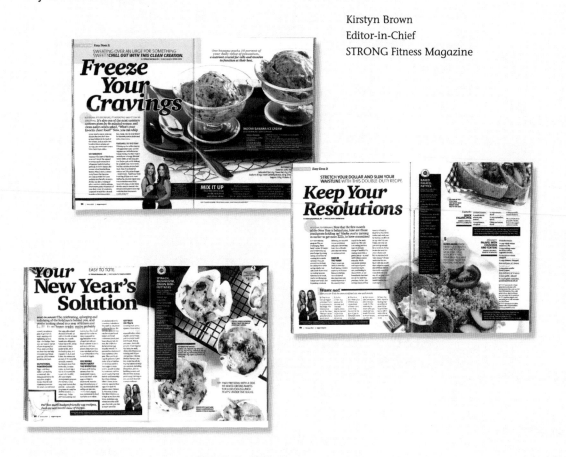

Introduction

The wisdom of our grandmother: Why we wrote this book

We grew up in the 70's, surrounded by processed foods, eating TV dinners, sugarcoated cereal and Wonder Bread. Macaroni and cheese was what we considered a food group. We had no idea that the chemically-processed junk foods were taking their toll on our bodies, wreaking havoc with our metabolism and immune systems.

However, our frequent visits to our grandmother's house always left us feeling noticeably more energetic, as a result of the natural foods she prepared. Grandma mixed love with fresh, seasonal ingredients which looked and tasted rich, colorful and succulent. These natural whole foods were more easily digested and our bodies thanked us by providing an overall sense of well-being. Our skin and bodies looked healthier. We glowed, and it showed. This fascinated both of us and was certainly one of the reasons we both wound up pursuing careers in the field of nutrition. We were learning, and we wanted to learn more. As our bodies craved the healthful nutrition, our minds craved more knowledge. Intellectually, we knew that our diet affected every aspect of our bodies. But as humans, we were realistic. We knew if the preparation was time-consuming or the result bland-tasting, we would never eat it. Our society has moved so far away from the way our ancestors

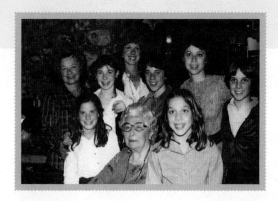

prepared food that our taste buds have become accustomed to additives, preservatives and chemicals.

The best way to a naturally lean, healthy body is to get back to the basics of eating clean and simple. You may ask, "Why a breakfast cookbook?" We strongly subscribe to the notion that breakfast is the most important meal of the day.

Some experts state the importance of "breaking the fast" after a night's sleep, noting that without this meal, a body will have problems with metabolism, weight, concentration and cardiac health. We find that when the body is given a nutritious, healthful, satiating meal, it is less likely to crave unhealthy snacks as the day progresses. Being mindful at breakfast leads to healthier meal choices throughout the day.

We've titled our book *"No Excuses: 50 Healthy Ways to ROCK Breakfast"* because we want you to know that eating healthful food can be fun as well as delicious. You'll also derive a much-added benefit of knowing that the tasty and nutritious foods you're preparing are helping your body stay strong and lean so you can be active, healthy and strong for yourself and your loved ones.

Here's to eating well, looking good and feeling fabulous!

Tiffani and Erin

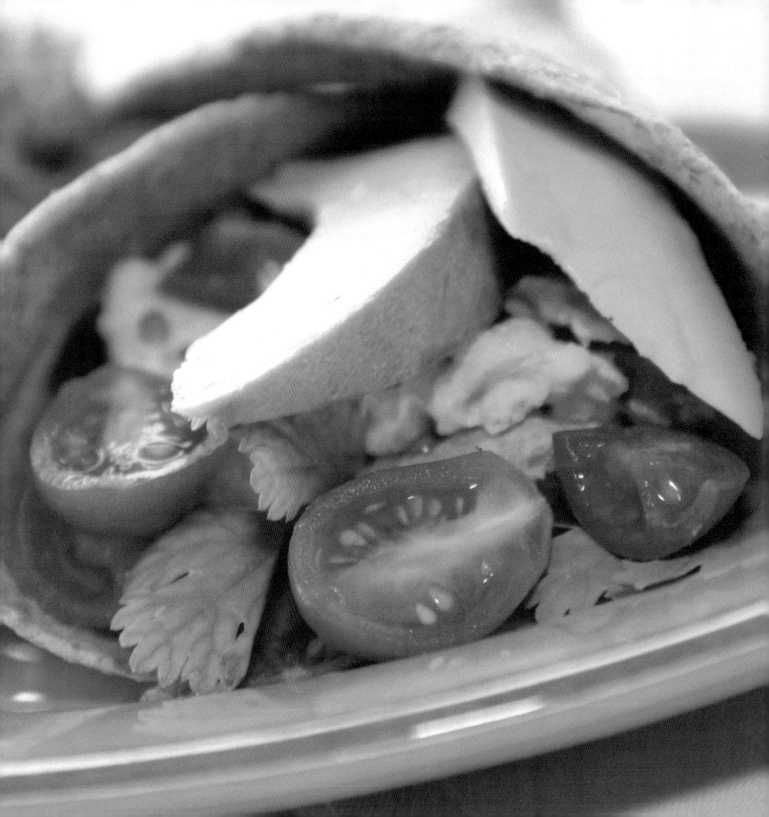

Welcome

to the No Excuses Zone

Despite knowing the importance of eating clean, process-free foods, we hear from our clients all of the time that it's too hard to eat well and nourish their bodies properly. "I don't have time," "It's too expensive," or "I don't know what to make" are just a few of the reasons that our clients give us on a daily basis.

Well, you have just entered a "no excuses" zone!

We've designed this cookbook to show you how to nourish your body properly, give it the food it craves and do so quickly and inexpensively. Say "goodbye" to excuses and "hello" to the body you deserve.

Many diet books offer quick fixes: "Lose 10 pounds in two weeks! Drop a dress size in five days!" While these diets may lead to short-term success, they're unsustainable over time. The weight often comes back as quickly as it came off. If you've been on one or more of these so-called "miracle" diets, you know this to be true.

Television programs like "The Biggest Loser" attract large audiences by showing participants adhering to strict diet and exercise plans and losing hundreds of pounds in the process. But what they don't show you is how the participants handle life when they are back in their real world environment. Without constant supervision, many regain the weight they have lost. Some contestants gain more than they originally lost.

Many people "go on a diet" or temporarily plan to lose weight. We believe that your "diet" is the food or drink consumed as nourishment. Therefore, the purpose of our book is not to offer another quick fix. We believe that there are no shortcuts when it comes to developing a healthy body. The solution is to make realistic and achievable changes that will become habitual and last a lifetime.

The straight scoop: changing your relationship with food

Our goal in writing this book is to give you the straight scoop on what it takes to develop and maintain a healthy lifestyle that stands the test of time. We offer a no-nonsense approach to healthful eating that can survive the daily ups and downs of life. Our goal is not to help you lose weight. Our goal is to help you to change your relationship with food. As a result of this change, you will lose weight . . . naturally.

So what do we mean when we say we want to change your relationship with food?

When we take an honest look at our lives, we can see that our days are filled with routines and habits, some of which we have been attached to for years. Much of what we do each day is rooted in our subconscious and we are unaware that we are constantly making choices.

Having choices means we have the opportunity to choose differently. We are not pre-destined to repeat today what we did yesterday. Yet, often times, we do.

We find ourselves reaching for the same snack at the same hour of day or driving into the same fast-food drive through day after day, week after week, year after year.

These learned behaviors are mostly a matter of ingrained habits. Many of these habits and routines have become ritual to us, and they are extremely hard to break. We may even feel like victims trapped in habits over which we believe we have no choice. The truth, however, is that we're constantly presented with an opportunity to behave differently. We can decide at any time to create new habits.

Making the unconscious conscious

Food is one of the trickiest habits to change because we tend to use food as more than just fuel for our bodies. We may reach for that afternoon candy bar when we're tired, or grab a handful of potato chips when we're bored, or reach for a quart of ice cream when we're lonely or stressed. We all do it at one time or another. It's tremendously difficult for us to use food solely for the purpose it was intended, as fuel for our bodies. One of the first steps to changing our behavior is by making the unconscious conscious. This means we begin to notice when we are reaching for food. Is it to fuel our bodies or to quell some inner hunger or emotional discomfort?

By becoming more aware of what we eat, when we eat and how we eat, we can become more mindful of our relationship with food, our bodies and ourselves.

So, as you read this book, we will offer tips and ideas on how to pay attention to what you are eating and why you are eating.

So, why a breakfast cookbook?

We've all heard that breakfast is the most important meal of the day. This is true for many reasons.

Not only does breakfast provide the fuel most of us need to carry us through the early part of our day, breakfast also sets the stage for the next 24 hours.

When we take the time to prepare a healthful, nurturing breakfast for our families, and ourselves, we are developing the best foundation possible for making healthy food choices the rest of the day.

We are committing to a healthy food habit right out of the gate.

Physically, this means we are less likely to crash later in the day and reach for sugar as quick fuel. Mentally and emotionally, it means we've chosen to start our day with a healthy choice, improving the chances that we'll continue to choose healthy foods throughout the day.

In writing this cookbook, we've included some of our favorite breakfast recipes as an answer to our favorite excuses.

If you are ready to change your body, it's time to get started.

No more excuses.

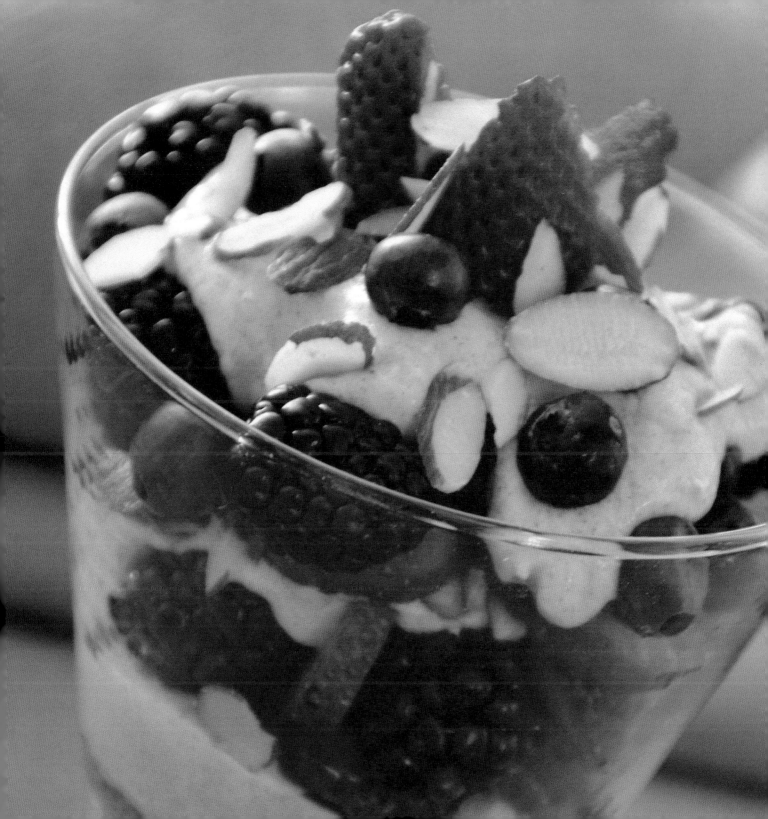

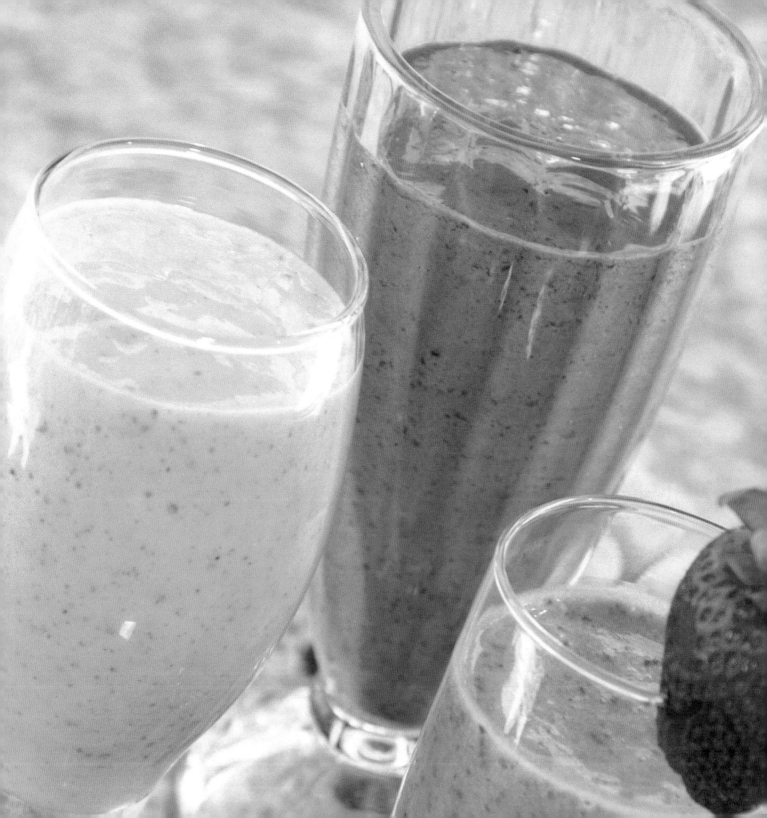

Chapter 2

"I Just Don't Have the Time"

Ok . . . We get it. Breakfast is not on your list of top priorities to add to your already busy, multi-tasking morning. Many people assume that making and eating breakfast is just too time-consuming and too cumbersome to be doable. The secret to finding time in the morning to make breakfast is pre-planning the night before. As you're winding down in the evening, think about the breakfast you'd like to have tomorrow. Then organize all of the ingredients you will need. When you wake up, you'll be ready to go.

Still not convinced? Think again! We've made this SIMPLE and EASY. These recipes were designed especially for YOU. Each takes less than 5 minutes to prepare in the morning. That's less time than you would spend in a drive-thru line.

Cinnamon Spice Cottage Cheese Toast

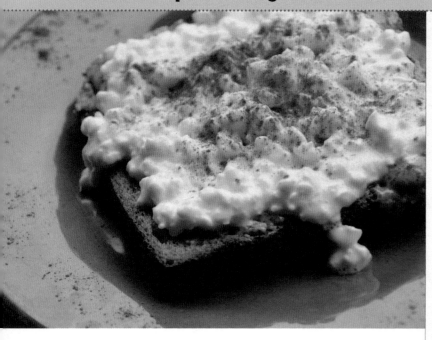

Makes 1 serving ~ Ready in less than 5 minutes

1 slice Ezekiel raisin bread
  or whole wheat bread
½ Tbsp. almond butter
½ cup of 1% cottage cheese
¼ tsp. of cinnamon

Directions:

1. Toast bread in toaster until lightly browned.
2. Spread on almond butter
3. Mix cottage cheese with cinnamon and spread on top of almond butter.

Nutrients per serving: 189 Calories, 7.1 g fat, 16.5 g Carbohydrates, 2.5 g fiber,

TIFF SAYS: *"I usually give this recipe to my clients on our first meeting because it's such a no-brainer and I always get rave reviews for its tasteful simplicity."*

ROCKIN' FACT Cinnamon helps control blood sugar level (which is great for weight loss) and is a great way to satisfy your sweet tooth without the calories. Cinnamon also helps with cognitive function and memory, lowers bad (LDL) cholesterol, and fights inflammation.

Much Ado about Muesli

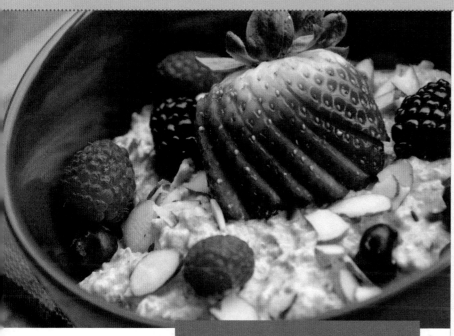

ROCKIN' FACT Steel cut oats take longer to digest than rolled oats, keeping you fuller for longer.

 TIFF SAYS: *"This recipe is a version of the popular muesli recipe we did for Oxygen Magazine's Easy Does It column (April, 2011)"*

Makes 1 serving ~ 5 min prep night before - 5 min prep in morning

½ cup rolled oats

¼ tsp. cinnamon

½ Tbsp. chia seed

½ cup nonfat plain Greek yogurt

½ cup unsweetened almond milk

⅛ tsp. almond extract

½ tsp. pure vanilla extract

1 Tbsp. 100% maple syrup
   (can substitute agave or date sugar)

½ cup seasonal, organic berries

2 Tbsp. sliced almonds

Directions:

1. In a bowl, combine oats, cinnamon, and chia seed. Add the yogurt, almond milk, almond and vanilla extracts and stir to combine.
2. Place bowl in refrigerator at least 6 hours, preferably overnight.
3. Remove bowl from refrigerator and add the berries and nuts and enjoy.

NUTRIENTS PER SERVING: **427** CALORIES, **13.1** G FAT, **58.7** G CARBOHYDRATES, **8.6** G FIBER, **23.1** G PROTEIN

Although this recipe makes one serving, you can easily double or triple and serve throughout the week.

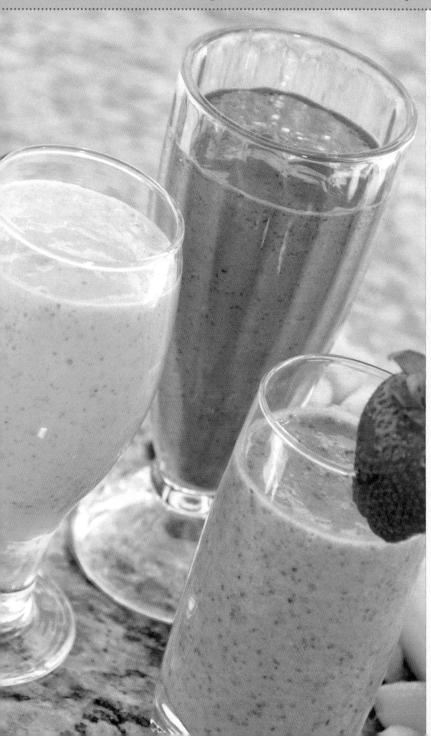

Mango Madness

*Makes 1 serving ~ Ready
in less than 5 minutes*

½ cup frozen mango

½ banana

6 oz. orange juice

4 oz. unsweetened vanilla almond milk

1 scoop vanilla whey vanilla
    protein powder

1 Tbsp. chia seed

- ice to desired consistency

NUTRIENTS PER SERVING: **371** CALORIES,
9.1 G FAT, **57.8** G CARBOHYDRATES,
8.9 G FIBER, **23.4** G PROTEIN

Bananaberry Bombshell

*Makes 1 serving ~ Ready
in less than 5 minutes*

¾ cup frozen strawberries

½ banana

6 oz. orange or tart cherry juice

1 scoop whey vanilla protein powder

1 Tbsp. chia seed

- ice to desired consistency

NUTRIENTS PER SERVING: 316 CALORIES,
5.0 G FAT, 50.2 G CARBOHYDRATES,
11.8 G FIBER, 24 G PROTEIN

Berry-licious

*Makes 1 serving ~ Ready
in less than 5 minutes*

¾ cup mixed berries

6 oz. tart cherry juice

1 scoop vanilla whey protein powder

1 Tbsp. chia seed

- ice to desired consistency

NUTRIENTS PER SERVING: 301 CALORIES,
4.5 G FAT, 43.5 G CARBOHYDRATES,
9.3 G FIBER, 24.3 G PROTEIN

 ERIN SAYS: *"My son Alex (14) is wild about the Mango Madness, while Ryan (16) prefers Berry-licious, and Eric (16) loves them all. It's such an easy after-school snack or breakfast-on-the-go."*

ROCKIN' FACT Chia seeds will help keep you fuller for longer and tart cherry juice helps fight muscle soreness and can improve your night's sleep without making you feel tired during the day.

Tropical Paradise Parfait

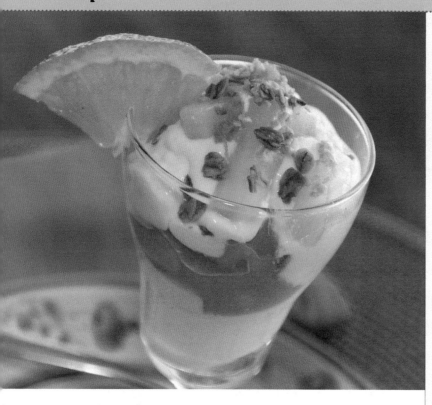

Makes 1 serving ~ Ready in less than 5 minutes

1 cup nonfat Greek yogurt

1 tsp. orange zest

1 tsp. vanilla extract

½ cup each chopped mango and pineapple

2 Tbsp. granola

Directions:

1. Combine the first three ingredients.
2. Place half of yogurt mixture in the bottom of a glass.
3. Add half of the fruit, then the granola.
4. Layer with the remaining yogurt, then top with mango and pineapple.

NUTRIENTS PER SERVING: 260 CALORIES, 0.6 G FAT, 53 G CARBOHYDRATES, 3 G FIBER, 13 G PROTEIN

ROCKIN' FACT Greek yogurt has more protein than regular yogurt, which will keep you energized and full for hours.

TIFF SAYS: *"This parfait has so many different flavors and textures that it really satisfies my need for something sweet, creamy, and crunchy."*

Cup o' Eggs

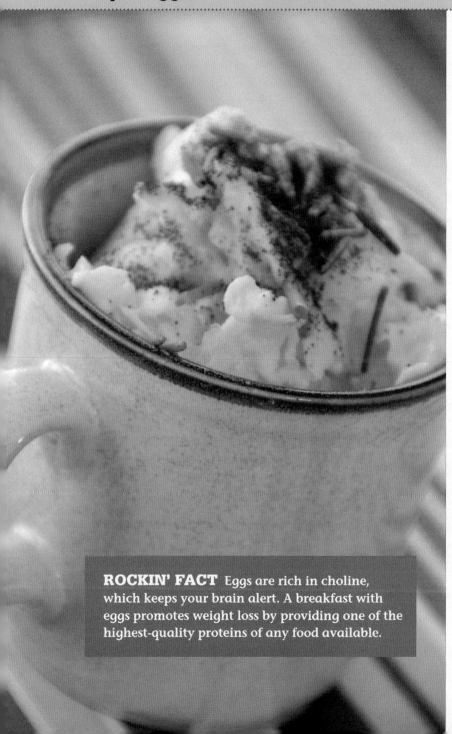

Makes 1 serving ~ Ready in less than 5 minutes

1 egg

½ Tbsp. Parmesan cheese

2 Tbsp. salsa (hot or mild)

Directions:

1. Whip up ingredients and place in a mug.
2. Cook for 60-90 seconds in microwave, until no liquid egg is observed underneath the egg.

NUTRIENTS PER SERVING: 95 CALORIES, 2.2 G FAT, 2.0 G CARBOHYDRATES, 1.0 G FIBER, 6.0 G PROTEIN

TIFF SAYS: *"This recipe is so great because I can make a different version of it every day. One day I might top it with salsa and guacamole, another day the cilantro pesto, and another day with a scoop of jam (trust me, it works)."*

ROCKIN' FACT Eggs are rich in choline, which keeps your brain alert. A breakfast with eggs promotes weight loss by providing one of the highest-quality proteins of any food available.

Bad-ass Burrito

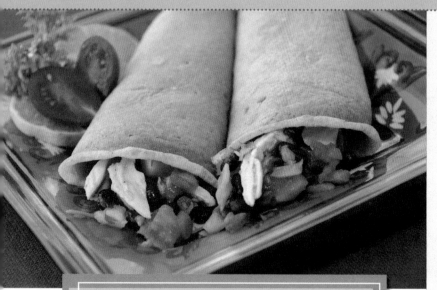

ERIN SAYS: *"I like to create a vegetarian version of this recipe by eliminating the chicken and adding black beans or some tofu. My kids still love the version with chicken because they feel it keeps them full longer at school."*

ROCKIN' FACT The healthy fat in avocado can make your skin appear moist and supple while keeping you full all morning long.

Makes 1 serving ~ 5 min prep night before - 5 min prep in morning

For those of you who don't like traditional breakfast foods, no one said you had to eat something that you'd find at the local diner or pancake house. Anything you like to eat will do, such as this black bean burrito. Packed with protein, smart carbs, and good fats, it will keep you full and feeling high-energy for hours.

1 (10-inch) whole wheat tortilla
⅓ cup black beans
3 oz. chicken
⅛ avocado slice
1 Tbsp. salsa (hot or mild)

Directions:

1. Lay the tortilla on a work surface. Add all of the ingredients and wrap up into a burrito. Wrap in foil and place in the refrigerator.
2. In the morning, remove from the fridge and take off the foil. Place on a plate and microwave for 1 minute to heat.

NUTRIENTS PER SERVING: 400 CALORIES, 9.7 G FAT, 45.6 G CARBOHYDRATES, 26.3 G FIBER, 32.2 G PROTEIN

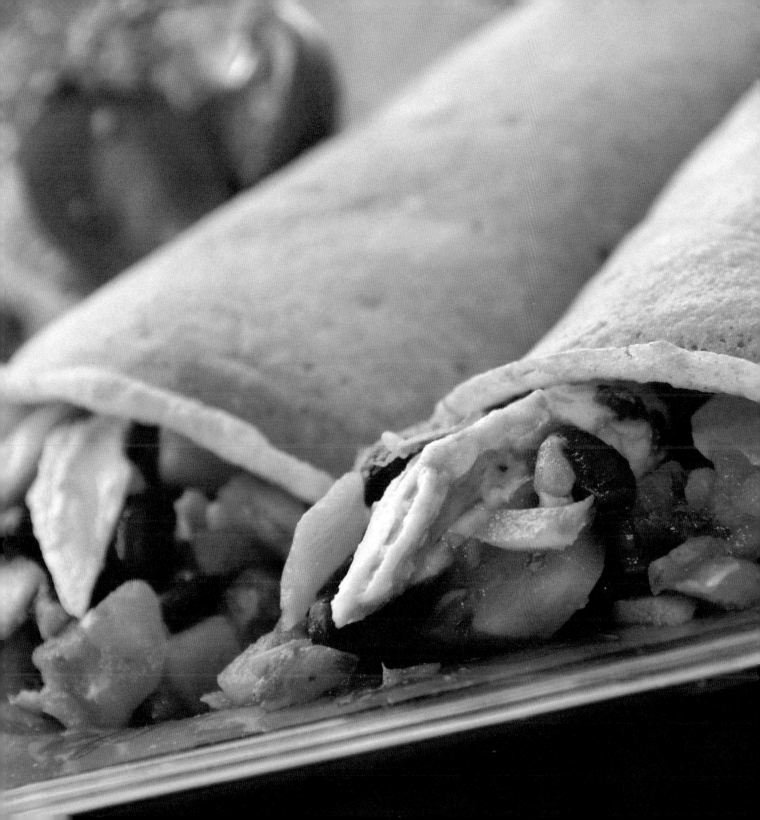

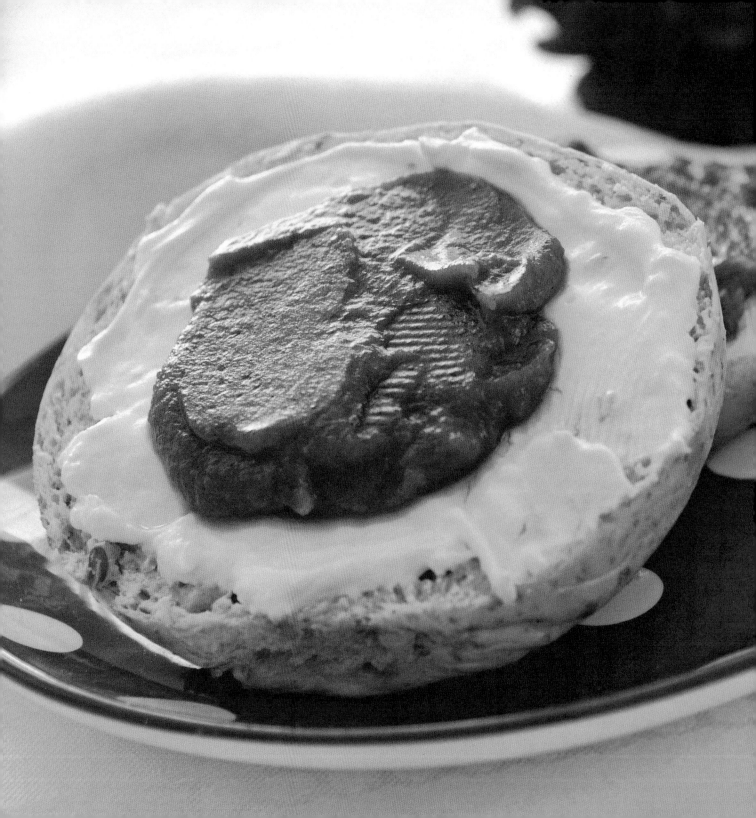

Chapter 3

"Eating Healthy Costs Too Much"

Planning healthy meals and buying fresh ingredients will actually save you money in the long run. Much of the cost of processed foods comes from the packaging. As you begin to buy food in its natural state more frequently, you will find your grocery bills going down, not up! The other nice thing about planning and cooking healthy meals is that you won't be tempted to stop by the nearest fast food place on your way home . . . a sure way to put a dent in your wallet!

We know there are a million things you'd rather spend your hard-earned money on. With these recipes, you don't need to buy expensive health food items. Save your money for a new bikini (because you're gonna need one).

Check out these budget-conscious breakfast recipes and see how they stack up to what's commercially available.

Egg Mac Muffin (compare to Egg McMuffin)

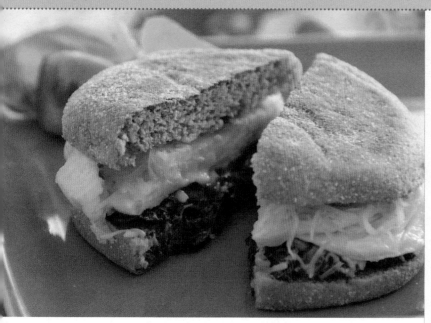

Makes 1 serving ~ Ready in less than 5 minutes

1 whole-grain English muffin
1 egg
2 Tbsp. cilantro pesto
  (see Extra Rockin' recipes page 88)
1 thin slice of fresh mozzarella cheese

Directions:

1. Place the English muffin in the toaster oven and cook until desired level of toastiness.
2. Coat a nonstick skillet with cooking spray and place over medium-high heat.
3. Whisk the egg in a bowl. Pour into the hot pan and scramble until cooked through.
4. Spread cilantro pesto on the bottom of the toasted English muffin. Place the scrambled egg on top of the pesto and then place the cheese on top of the egg. Place the other half of the English muffin on top of the cheese.

Cost $0.94
NUTRIENTS PER SERVING: 305 CALORIES, 11.8 G FAT, 29.1 G CARBOHYDRATES, 4.5 G FIBER, 20.2 G PROTEIN

COMPARED TO: McDonald's Egg McMuffin
COST $3.12
300 CALORIES, 12 G FAT, 32 G CARBOHYDRATES, 4 G FIBER, 18 G PROTEIN

ERIN SAYS: *"With a last name like Macdonald, people have always made reference to McDonald's. I figured I had to create a healthier version of their most popular breakfast sandwich; it didn't take long to come up with a tasty and healthier alternative."*

Bagel and Homemade Cream Cheese and 15-minute Pumpkin Butter

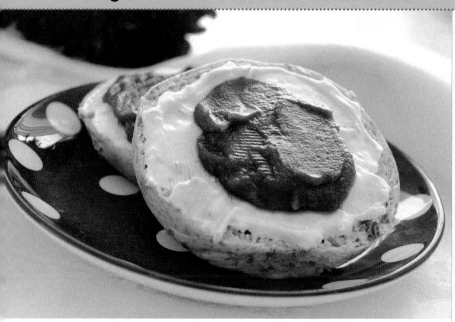

ERIN SAYS: *"The pumpkin butter is totally addictive. I love to eat it off the spoon when I'm craving something sweet to eat."*

COMPARED TO: bagel and cream cheese

Makes 1 serving ~

1 sprouted grain or whole wheat bagel

2 Tbsp. yogurt cheese
  (see Extra Rockin' Recipes, page 89)

2 Tbsp. pumpkin butter
  (see Extra Rockin' Recipes, page 90)

Directions:

1. Toast bagel and spread each half with 1 Tbsp. yogurt cheese and 1 Tbsp. pumpkin butter.

Cost $0.80

NUTRIENTS PER SERVING: **339** CALORIES, **1** G FAT, **67.2** G CARBOHYDRATES, **5.3** G FIBER, **16.1** G PROTEIN

COMPARED TO: Starbucks Multi-grain Bagel with Cream Cheese

COST: *$1.75*

430 CARBOHYDRATES, **14** G FAT, **64** G CARBOHYDRATES, **6** G FIBER, **17** G PROTEIN

Triple T (Totally Terrific Taco)

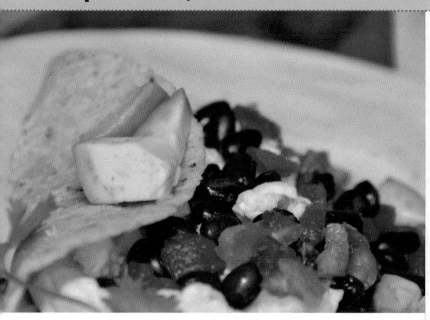

Makes 1 serving ~ Total time: 3 minutes

1 egg

3 Tbsp. salsa verde

2 tsp. Parmesan cheese

1 corn tortilla

- cilantro

- avocado

1 Tbsp. black beans

Directions:

1. Whisk salsa and egg.
   Mix in 2 tsp. cheese.

2. Warm the tortilla in the microwave
   for 30 seconds as you preheat a skillet.

3. Add eggs to pan and scramble for
   about 2 minutes.

4. Place mixture inside the tortilla, top-
   ping with the remaining ingredients.

Cost: $1.74

NUTRIENTS PER SERVING: 183 CALORIES,
9.8 G FAT, 15.8 G CARBOHYDRATES, 3.6 G FIBER,
9.4 G PROTEIN

COMPARED TO: Chicken Sausage Breakfast Wrap
COST: $3.25
300 CALORIES, 10 G FAT, 33 G CARBOHYDRATES,
4 G FIBER, 8 G PROTEIN

TIFF SAYS: *"Living in Arizona, we eat a lot of Mexican food. My kids love having Taco Tuesday, when we do tacos for breakfast and then again for dinner."*

PB&J Yogurt Parfait

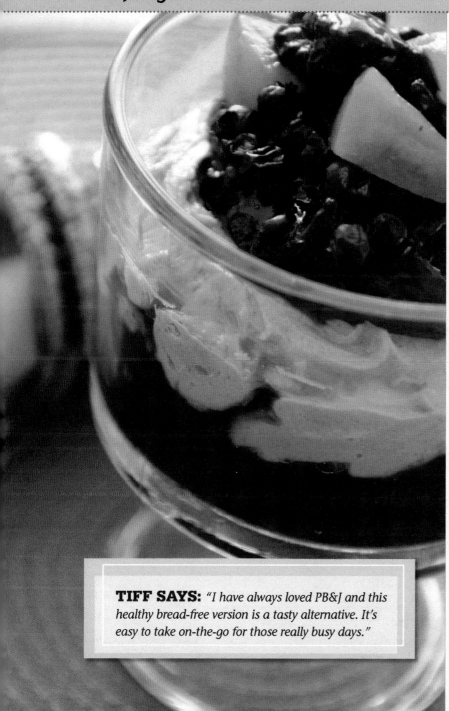

Makes 1 serving ~

½ Tbsp. all-natural peanut
  or almond butter
½ cup chia jam or other fruit compote
  (see Extra Rockin' Recipes, page 86, 87)
½ cup nonfat plain yogurt
½ tsp. vanilla extract
3 dashes cinnamon

Directions:

1. In a small bowl, combine the yogurt, almond butter, vanilla, and cinnamon.
2. Place ⅓ of the jam in a bottom of a glass. Add half of the yogurt mixture. Continue to alternate with a layer of jam, a layer of yogurt, and a layer of jam.

Cost: $1.72
NUTRIENTS PER SERVING: 312 CALORIES,
14.1 G FAT, 39.4 G CARBOHYDRATES,
14.8 G FIBER, 13 G PROTEIN
(USING STRAWBERRY CHIA JAM)

COMPARED TO: Starbucks parfait
COST: $3.45
290 CALORIES, 3.5 G FAT,
55 G CARBOHYDRATES, 4 G FIBER, 8 G PROTEIN

TIFF SAYS: *"I have always loved PB&J and this healthy bread-free version is a tasty alternative. It's easy to take on-the-go for those really busy days."*

Rockin' Banana Mocha Whip

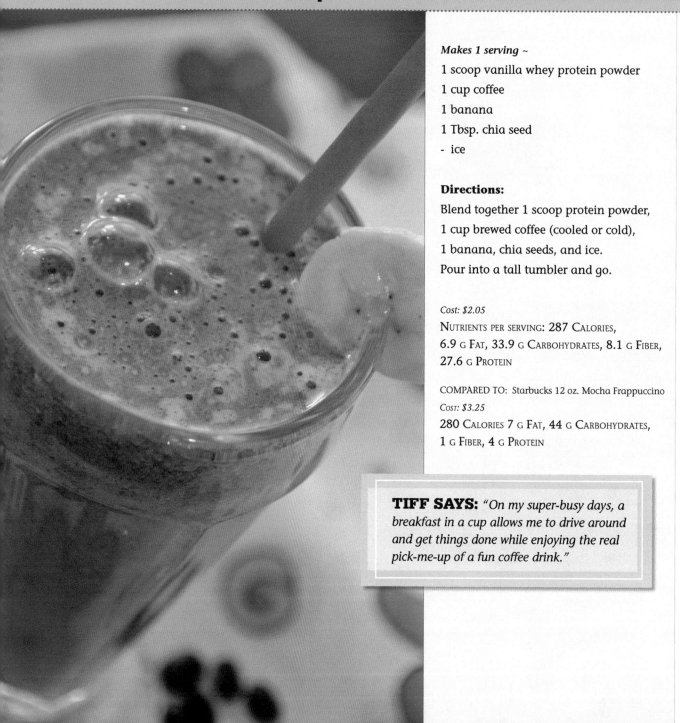

Makes 1 serving ~

1 scoop vanilla whey protein powder

1 cup coffee

1 banana

1 Tbsp. chia seed

- ice

Directions:

Blend together 1 scoop protein powder,
1 cup brewed coffee (cooled or cold),
1 banana, chia seeds, and ice.
Pour into a tall tumbler and go.

Cost: $2.05

NUTRIENTS PER SERVING: 287 CALORIES,
6.9 G FAT, 33.9 G CARBOHYDRATES, 8.1 G FIBER,
27.6 G PROTEIN

COMPARED TO: Starbucks 12 oz. Mocha Frappuccino

Cost: $3.25

280 CALORIES 7 G FAT, 44 G CARBOHYDRATES,
1 G FIBER, 4 G PROTEIN

TIFF SAYS: *"On my super-busy days, a
breakfast in a cup allows me to drive around
and get things done while enjoying the real
pick-me-up of a fun coffee drink."*

Chock Full of Bananas Mini Muffins

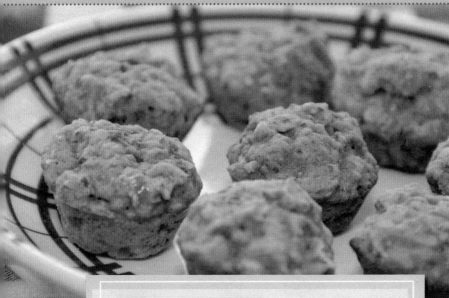

TIFF SAYS: *"I love to grab a muffin on the way to my workout because it gives me a quick burst of energy (check out more pre-and post-workout meal and snack ideas in Chapter 7)."*

Makes 24 mini muffins ~
Serving size 3 muffins

1 ¼ cup whole wheat pastry flour

2 tsp. baking powder

- Pinch salt

2 large or 3 small very ripe bananas

1 egg

¼ cup agave nectar

½ tsp. ground cinnamon

1 tsp. vanilla extract

1 Tbsp. chia seed

1 Tbsp. ground flax seed

Directions:

1. Preheat oven to 350°F.
2. In a medium bowl, combine flour, baking powder, and salt. Whisk to combine.
3. In a large mixing bowl, mash the banana with the egg, agave, cinnamon, vanilla extract, chia seed, and flax seed; mix well. Add the dry ingredients to the wet ingredients and gently stir to combine. Do not over mix!
4. Spray a mini-muffin tin with canola oil cooking spray. Use a small ice cream scoop to fill the muffin tray and then place in the oven.
5. Bake for 12 minutes or until light golden color on top.
6. Remove from oven and let cool 5 minutes in pan; remove and place on baking rack to cool completely.
7. Best served warm!

Cost: $0.27 per serving
NUTRIENTS PER SERVING: **153** CALORIES, **1.7** G FAT, **31.9** G CARBOHYDRATES, **4.4** G FIBER, **3.6** G PROTEIN

COMPARED TO: Starbucks Banana Walnut Bread
COST: *$2.75*
490 CALORIES, **19** G FAT, **75** G CARBOHYDRATES, **4** G FIBER, **7** G PROTEIN

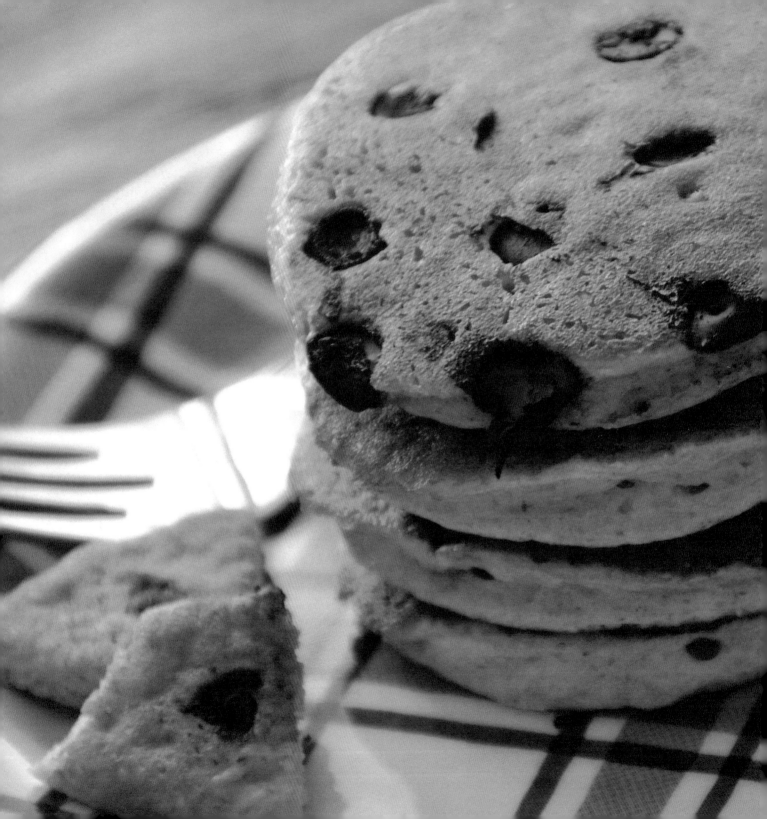

Chapter 4

"I Don't Want to be a Short Order Cook"

. . . and have to cook a different breakfast for every member of my family!

Attention, moms! Do you have picky kids? Are you tired of making a separate breakfast for EVERYONE in the house? With these recipes, you won't have to. The secret to these recipes is that they're both tasty and pack a healthy punch. So watch your kids scramble to the breakfast table for these sumptuous dishes. (Just don't tell them that it's healthy!)

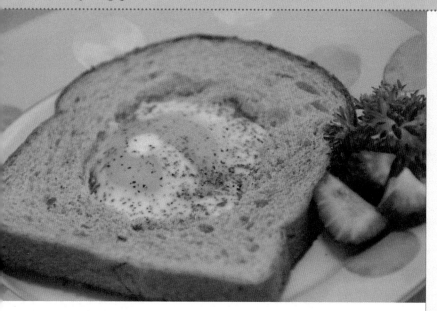

Makes 4 servings ~ Total time: 4 minutes

4 slices whole-grain bread (or sprouted grain, or Gluten Free whole grain bread)

4 eggs

- smoked paprika
- cooking spray

Directions:

1. Cut a hole out of bread and place in sprayed skillet.
2. Crack egg, drop directly into hole, sprinkle with some smoked paprika and cook for 60-90 seconds.
3. Flip and cook an additional 30 - 60 seconds, depending on how runny or well-cooked you prefer the yolk.

NUTRIENTS PER SERVING: 143 CALORIES, 6.4 G FAT, 14.3 G CARBOHYDRATES, 3.0 G FIBER, 9.5 G PROTEIN

ROCKIN' FACT Because sprouted grain bread has no preservatives, make sure to keep it in the refrigerator or freezer so it stays fresh for longer.

ERIN SAYS: *"My son Alex loves this recipe because he likes to soak up the crunchy bread with the runny egg yolk. It's pretty cool to watch how happy it makes him!"*

Chocolate Monkey Muffins

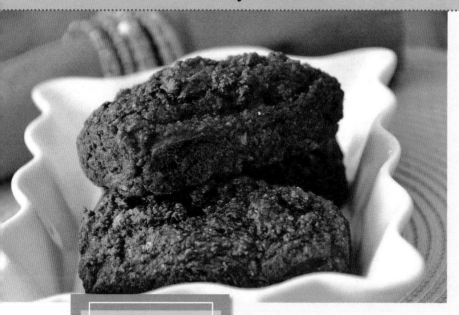

ERIN SAYS:

"Some mornings are so busy that I whip up the batter at night and place in a covered container in the refrigerator. In the morning I just heat up the oven, scoop out the batter and fresh muffins are on the table in less than 20 minutes."

Makes 12 muffins ~

1 ¼ cup whole wheat pastry flour

2 tsp. baking powder

3 Tbsp. dark cocoa powder

pinch salt

2 large or 3 small very ripe bananas

1 egg

¼ cup agave nectar or honey

½ tsp. ground cinnamon

1 tsp. vanilla extract

1 Tbsp. chia seed

1 Tbsp. ground flax seed

Directions:

1. Preheat oven to 350°F.
2. In a medium bowl, combine flour, baking powder, cocoa powder, and salt. Whisk to combine.
3. In a large mixing bowl, mash the banana with the egg, agave, cinnamon, vanilla extract, chia seed, and flax seed; mix well. Add the dry ingredients to the wet ingredients and gently stir to combine. Do not overmix!
4. Spray a muffin tin with canola oil cooking spray. Use a ½-cup measuring cup to fill each muffin hole and then place in the oven. Bake for 18 minutes or until light golden color on top.
5. Remove from oven and let cool 5 minutes in pan; remove and place on baking rack to cool completely.
6. Best served warm! This also can be done in a loaf pan or an 8-inch glass baking dish and tell your kids it's "cake!" Dessert never was so healthy!

NUTRIENTS PER SERVING: 105 CALORIES, 1.3 G FAT, 21.6 G CARBOHYDRATES, 3.8 G FIBER, 2.61 G PROTEIN

ROCKIN' FACT Dark cocoa powder gives you all the chocolaty goodness without all the calories and fat of chocolate. Plus it's high in antioxidants, which means it's good for you!

Nutty Maple Apple Oatmeal (crockpot)

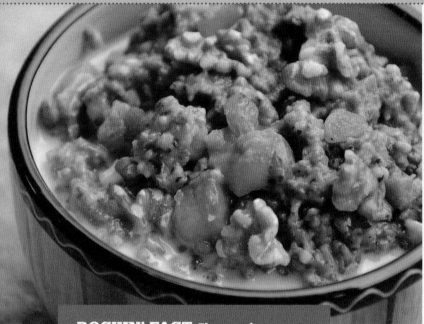

*Makes 7 (3/4 c) servings ~ Prep 5 minutes
at night – Ready in the morning*
*Makes enough to feed your whole family or
breakfast for the single gal for the whole week.*

2 apples, peeled and chopped into ½ inch
    pieces (Fuji, Pink Lady, or Granny Smith)
1 ½ cup unsweetened vanilla almond milk
1 ½ cup water
1 cup steel cut oats
2 Tbsp. maple syrup
¼ cup golden raisins
1 tsp. cinnamon
2 Tbsp. ground flax seed
2 Tbsp. chia seed
¼ tsp. sea salt
Add-on in the morning: ¼ cup chopped
pecans or walnuts

ROCKIN' FACT Flax seeds can go
rancid quickly, so buy them whole and
grind them yourself. Keep the seeds in
the refrigerator to preserve freshness.

TIFF SAYS: *"This dish screams
'comfort food'! My whole house smells
insanely delicious when I cook this recipe."*

Directions:

1. Coat the inside of a 3 ½-qt (or larger)
   slow cooker with canola oil cooking
   spray. Add all ingredients (except nuts)
   to slow cooker and stir to combine.
   Cover and cook on low for 7 hours.
   (Your crock pot will keep it warm until
   you wake up; it won't over cook.)

2. To reheat for another day, scoop out
   your portion of oatmeal and add
   some more unsweetened almond milk
   and reheat in the microwave.

NUTRITION FACTS WITHOUT ADD-ONS:
190 CALORIES, 4.3 G FAT,
33.7 G CARBOHYDRATES, 7 G FIBER, 5.5 G PROTEIN

WITH ADD-ONS (CHOPPED PECANS):
219 CALORIES, 7.3 G FAT,
34.3 G CARBOHYDRATES, 7.3 G FIBER, 5.9 G PROTEIN

Chocolate Chip Pancakes

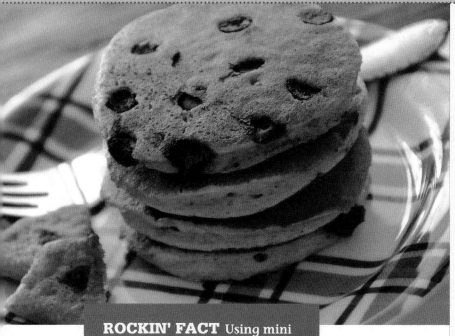

ROCKIN' FACT Using mini chocolate chips is a great way to get more chocolate in every bite without racking up the calories.

TIFF SAYS: *"This is a perfect Saturday morning recipe because it's the one day we can all sit around and have breakfast together. It's my son Dylan's (14) favorite breakfast before a basketball game.*

Makes 8 pancakes ~ Serving size 2 pancakes

3 eggs (2 egg whites + 1 egg)

¼ cup unsweetened rice milk or unsweetened vanilla almond milk

¾ cup old-fashioned rolled oats (dry uncooked)

1 tsp. baking powder

⅓ cup low-fat cottage cheese

1 tsp. honey (preferably raw)

1 scoop vanilla protein powder (whey or plant)

1 Tbsp. unrefined coconut oil

¼ cup mini, semi-sweet chocolate chips

Directions:

1. Place all ingredients (except chocolate chips) in a blender and blend until smooth. Pour into a bowl and fold in chocolate chips.

2. Heat a nonstick pan or griddle over medium-high heat. Add 1 Tbsp. unrefined coconut oil to pan. When it melts and is hot, ladle 2 Tbsp. of batter onto griddle. Let cook 2-3 minutes, or until light golden color develops on bottom; flip and cook another 2-3 minutes. Repeat with remaining batter.

NUTRIENTS PER SERVING: 191 CALORIES, 6.9 G FAT, 20 G CARBOHYDRATES, 1 G FIBER, 13 G PROTEIN

Apple-Cinnamon Raisin Bread Pudding with Maple "Cream"

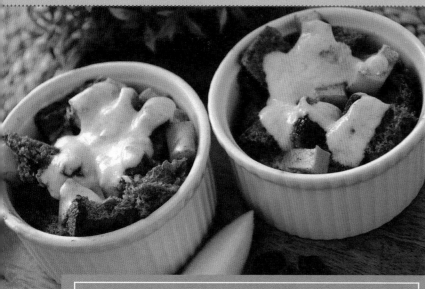

ERIN SAYS: *"Our family loves the combination of apples and cinnamon. It just warms your soul. You can substitute peaches in the summer or pears in the fall for the apples."*

Makes 4 servings ~

2 apples (Fuji or Granny Smith), chopped

1 tsp. cinnamon

4 slices Ezekiel raisin bread, cut into chunks

2 eggs or ½ cup egg beaters

2 Tbsp. agave or honey

½ cup milk

- dash vanilla

1 tsp. virgin coconut oil, melted

1 Tbsp. chia seeds

1 cup nonfat plain yogurt

1 Tbsp. pure maple syrup

¼ tsp. cinnamon

Directions:

1. Preheat oven to 350°F. Prepare an 8-inch baking dish by coating it with cooking spray or coconut oil.
2. Place apples, cinnamon, and bread in a large bowl. In another bowl, whisk together eggs, agave, milk, vanilla extract, melted coconut oil, and chia seeds. Pour over bread mixture and let soak 30 minutes.
3. Pour soaked bread mixture into baking dish and place in oven. Bake 25 minutes.
4. While bread pudding is cooking, whisk together the yogurt, maple syrup, and cinnamon.
5. Remove bread pudding from oven and let cool 10 minutes before serving. Scoop out bread pudding into bowls and top with a generous scoop of maple cream.

NUTRIENTS PER SERVING: **285** CALORIES, **6.7** G FAT, **47.9** G CARBOHYDRATES, **6.4** G FIBER, **10.8** G PROTEIN

ROCKIN' FACT Make sure to buy organic apples, as they are one of the "Dirty Dozen" – most highly sprayed with pesticides

Breakfast Pizza

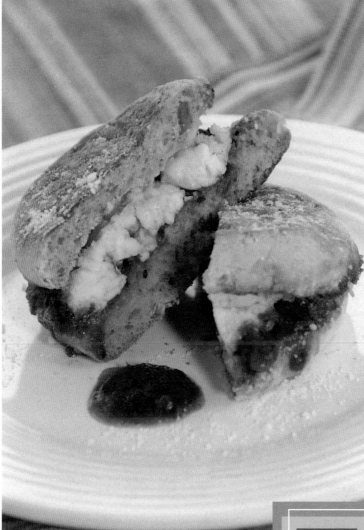

Makes 4 servings ~

4 whole grain or sprouted grain
   English muffins
1 cup organic marinara sauce
4 eggs, scrambled
4 Tbsp. parmesan cheese

Directions:

1. Preheat oven to broil. Make sure the oven rack is approximately 6 inches away from the heating element.
2. Split each muffin in half and place on a baking sheet. Place marinara sauce on each muffin half. Top with scrambled egg and parmesan cheese. Place under the broiler in oven and cook until cheese starts to turn golden brown, about 1-2 minutes.
3. Serve 2 muffin halves.

NUTRIENTS PER SERVING: **288** CALORIES,
11.2 G FAT, **32.6** G CARBOHYDRATES,
6.5 G FIBER, **16.5** G PROTEIN

ROCKIN' FACT Parmesan cheese packs a big flavor punch for very few calories

ERIN SAYS: *"My kids love pizza (who doesn't?) and breakfast pizza is an easy sell on a school morning. Plus it gives them all the nutrition they need so they can stay focused in class."*

Pancakes with Mixed Berry Compote

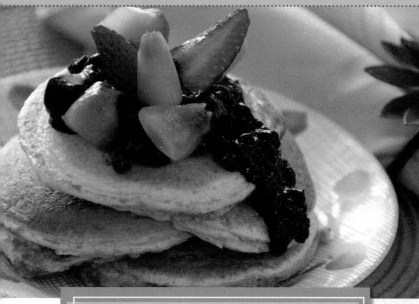

1 Tbsp. honey

½ tsp. ground cinnamon

2 cups berry compote

(see Extra Rockin' Recipes, page 86)

Directions:

1. Mix all dry ingredients together in a bowl; add all wet ingredients and stir to combine. Let sit for 5 minutes. If too thick, add a little more almond milk.

2. Heat a large nonstick pan over medium-high heat and add ½ Tbsp. canola oil or coconut oil. When the pan is hot, add batter (2 Tbsp. for mini pancakes or ¼ cup for medium pancakes). Cook about 2-3 minutes, or until golden on bottom; flip and cook 2-3 minutes or until golden.

3. Serve with berry compote on top.

NUTRIENTS PER SERVING: 314 CALORIES, 4.6 G FAT, 63.5 G CARBOHYDRATES, 8.4 G FIBER, 7.7 G PROTEIN

ERIN SAYS: *"My family loves this berry compote because it can also be used as a delicious dessert. I just heat it and top with a dollop of nonfat vanilla or lemon Greek yogurt."*

Makes 4 servings ~

1 cup whole wheat pastry flour

½ cup old-fashioned oats

1 tsp. baking powder

½ tsp. baking soda

2 Tbsp. ground flax seed

1 Tbsp. chia seed

1-½ cup unsweetened vanilla almond milk

¼ cup nonfat plain Greek yogurt

1 tsp. vanilla extract

ROCKIN' FACT Berries are low in calories and high in fiber which can help you lose those last few stubborn pounds.

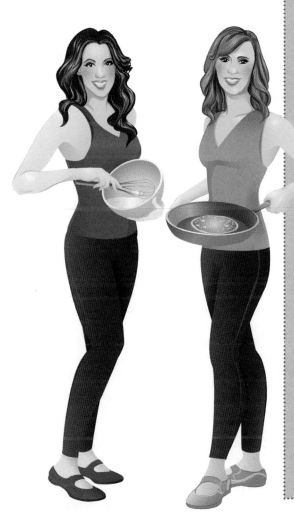

ROCKIN' FACTS
from Tiffani and Erin

ROCKIN' FACT Date sugar is a high-fiber, mineral rich sugar that is much sweeter than sugar, so less can be used when substituting it in your recipes. 1 tablespoon. date sugar has 33 calories (compared to 45 calories in sugar, and 60 in agave and honey). If you can't find date sugar in your local health food store, just substitute honey, maple syrup, or agave.

ROCKIN' FACT Consuming whey protein as part of a nutritious diet can help aid in weight-loss efforts.

ROCKIN' FACT Tart cherry juice helps fight muscle soreness and can improve your night's sleep (it won't make you sleepy during the day).

ROCKIN' FACT Chia seeds will help keep you fuller for longer.

ROCKIN' FACT Corn tortillas are gluten-free, a great substitute if you are gluten sensitive or have Celiac disease.

ROCKIN' FACT Coffee is actually good for you! It can speed up your metabolism (hello weight loss!), help you body burn more fat while exercising, and keep you more focused (so you can stay on task during the work day).

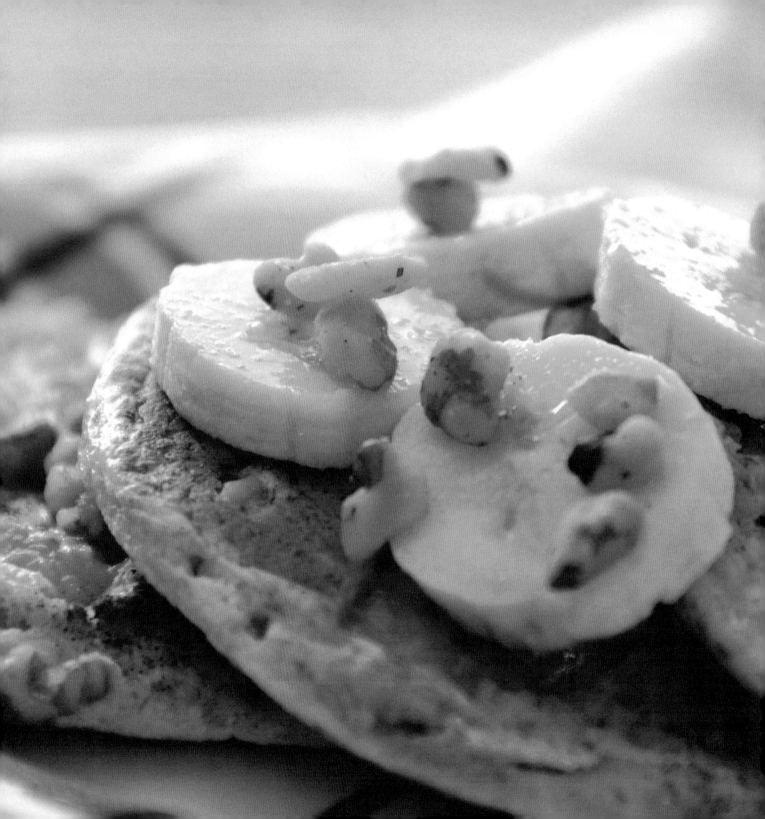

Chapter 5

"Carbs Make Me Fat"

Many people falsely accuse carbs of being the weight loss enemy. The most important thing to remember is that you need to balance your carbs with protein at each meal. A breakfast that is too heavy in carbs like a bagel with cream cheese or a blueberry muffin will spike your blood sugar and then crash you back down, making you crave even more carbs. However, studies show that eating a protein-rich breakfast that includes carbs helps with weight loss and weight management, as well as control of carb cravings. Protein + carbs (high-fiber carbs such as vegetables and fruit) at breakfast keep you fuller for longer. So don't be afraid to include a healthy dose of minimally-processed carbs – preferably of the whole food variety – in every meal.

Smashing Southwestern Sweet Potato Hash

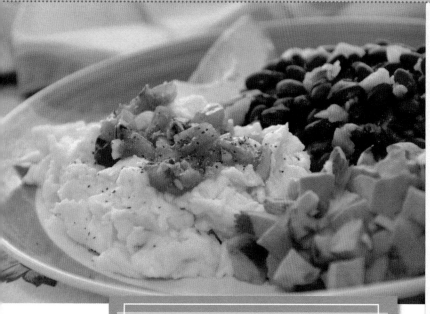

> **ERIN SAYS:** *"My clients find that when they eat more for breakfast, they eat better the rest of the day. This breakfast will keep you full – and full of energy – for hours!"*

ROCKIN' FACT Sweet potatoes in their whole, natural state, are considered a "clean carb" because they breakdown slower than processed carbs, giving you a steady stream of energy.

Makes 2 servings ~ Total time: 10 minutes

Sweet Potato Hash

1 small sweet potato, diced or shredded

3 Tbsp. onion, chopped

½ link chicken apple sausage, cut into small pieces

¼ tsp. fresh cilantro, chopped

Directions:

1. Coat a nonstick skillet with cooking spray and place over medium-high heat until hot. Add sweet potato, onion and sausage to pan with a pinch of sea salt and cook until golden so that the sweet flavors can develop.
2. Add cilantro and cook for about 30 seconds longer. Divide between 2 plates.

Scrambled Eggs and Salsa

6 egg whites

2 Tbsp. chunky salsa (your choice of hot or mild)

Directions:

1. Coat a nonstick skillet with cooking spray and place over medium-high heat until hot. Add egg whites and cook until set on the bottom; flip and cook 30 seconds.
2. Divide in half and transfer to 2 plates. Top with salsa.

Green Chile Black beans

⅔ cup black beans (canned, rinsed
   and drained)

2 Tbsp. diced green chilies
   (such as Ortega brand)

⅛ avocado, sliced

Directions:

1. Stir together beans and chilies and
   heat in microwave or on stove until
   hot. Divide among plates with hash
   and eggs and top with avocado slices.

NUTRIENTS PER SERVING: 147 CALORIES,
3.7 G FAT, 18.9 G CARBOHYDRATES,
3.1 G FIBER, 9.5 G PROTEIN

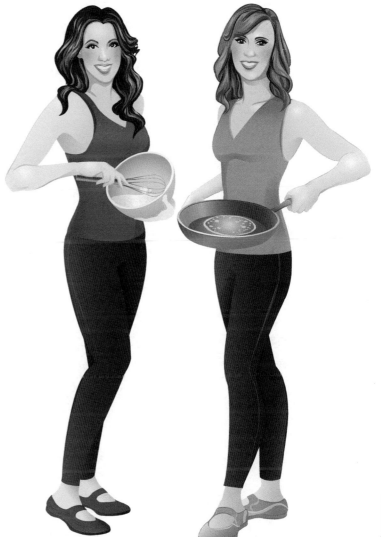

Tofu Parfait

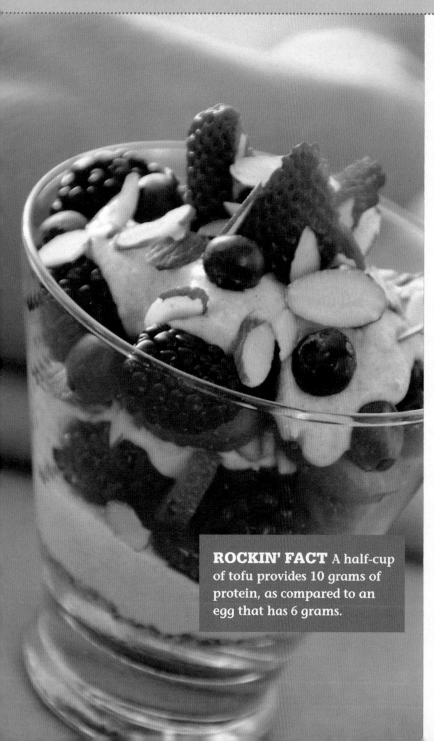

ROCKIN' FACT A half-cup of tofu provides 10 grams of protein, as compared to an egg that has 6 grams.

Makes 2 servings ~

12 oz. soft silken tofu (non-GMO)

2 tsp. honey (preferably raw)

1 tsp. vanilla extract

1 tsp. cinnamon

1 tsp. orange zest

1 cup mixed fresh berries

4 tsp. ground flaxseed

4 tsp. raw almond halves (crushed)

Directions:

1. In blender mix tofu, honey, vanilla extract, cinnamon and orange zest until smooth.

2. In a small bowl, mix ground flaxseed and almonds.

3. Take 2 serving cups or bowls and place on the counter. Fill each cup with half of the flax/almond mixture followed by half of the tofu mixture and top with half of the berries.

NUTRIENTS PER SERVING: **187** CALORIES, **8.8** G FAT, **20.3** G CARBOHYDRATES, **4.3** G FIBER, **10.3** G PROTEIN

TIFF SAYS: *"My daughter Riley (7) loves this for breakfast and for an after-school snack and it's so easy to make that she can do it by herself (under my watchful eye)."*

Peanut Butter and Banana Shake

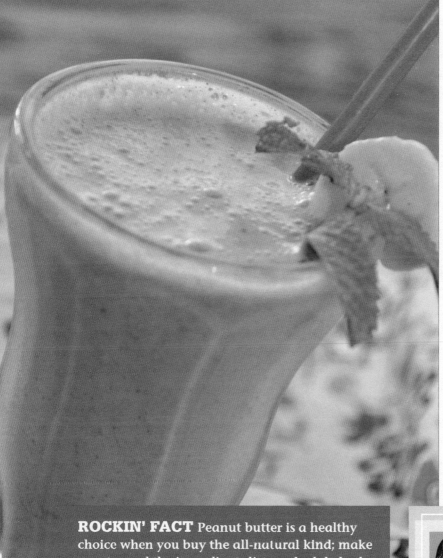

Makes 1 serving ~

1 scoop vanilla protein powder

1 Tbsp. all-natural peanut butter

1 banana (frozen)

1 cup unsweetened vanilla almond milk

- ice (if necessary)

Directions:

1. Place all of the ingredients, except for the ice, into a blender and blend until smooth.
2. Add the ice, a few cubes at a time, until the desired consistency is reached.

NUTRIENTS PER SERVING: **330** CALORIES, **11.4** G FAT, **35.5** G CARBOHYDRATES, **4.6** G FIBER, **26.3** G PROTEIN

ROCKIN' FACT Peanut butter is a healthy choice when you buy the all-natural kind; make sure to read the ingredients list on the label - the only ingredients should be peanuts and salt. Of course, if you can't have peanuts, feel free to substitute any other nut butter.

TIFF SAYS: *"This simple, easy and tasty breakfast (also works well for a snack or post-workout meal) keeps me satiated until my next meal."*

Banana Walnut Protein Pancakes

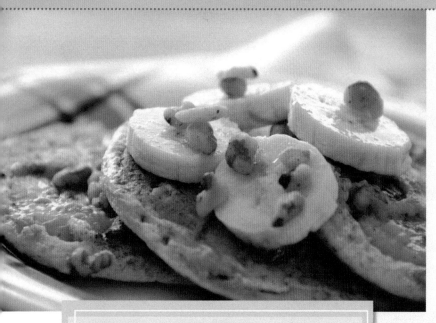

½ banana slices
⅓ cup raw walnut pieces
Cinnamon to taste

Directions:

1. Place all ingredients (except bananas, walnuts and cinnamon) in a blender and blend until smooth.
   Pour into a bowl and fold in walnuts.

2. Heat a nonstick pan or griddle over medium-high heat. Add 1 Tbsp. unrefined coconut oil to pan. When it melts and is hot, ladle 2 Tbsp. of batter onto griddle.

3. Add sliced bananas on top of each pancake with a sprinkle of cinnamon. Let cook 2-3 minutes, or until light golden color develops on bottom; flip and cook another 2-3 minutes. Repeat with remaining batter.

NUTRIENTS PER SERVING: 243 CALORIES, 12.9 G FAT, 18.3 G CARBOHYDRATES, 2.9 G FIBER, 13.9 G PROTEIN

TIFF SAYS: *"These recipes where I throw everything in a blender are my favorite because they're so darn easy. There is very little mess which means very little clean-up."*

Makes 8 pancakes ~ Serving size 2 pancakes
3 eggs (2 egg whites + 1 egg)
¼ cup unsweetened rice milk or unsweetened vanilla almond milk
¾ cup old-fashioned rolled oats (dry uncooked)
1 tsp. baking powder
⅓ cup low-fat cottage cheese
1 tsp. honey (preferably raw)
1 scoop vanilla whey protein powder
1 Tbsp. unrefined coconut oil

ROCKIN' FACT Walnuts are a great plant-source of those anti-inflammatory omega-3s you need to be getting more of in your diet.

Spinach, Mushroom, Onion Omelet

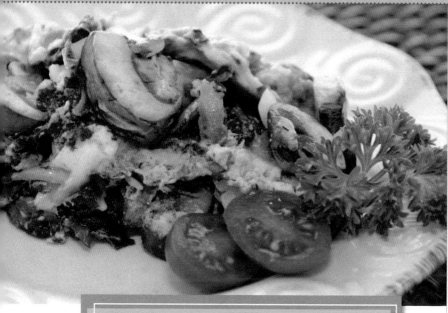

Makes 1 serving ~

4 egg whites

1 cup baby spinach leaves

3 Tbsp. chopped onion

½ cup chopped mushrooms

Directions:

1. Heat a nonstick pan and coat with cooking spray. When hot, add the mushrooms and onion and sauté with a pinch of sea salt and pepper for approximately 2 minutes. Add spinach and cook until wilted, about 1 minute.

2. Meanwhile, whisk the eggs, pour on top of the vegetables and cook for 1 minute.

3. Add the Parmesan, then flip and let cook about 1 minute more.

4. Fold in half and cook 30 seconds. Flip and cook for 30 more seconds on the remaining side.

NUTRIENTS PER SERVING: 121 CALORIES, 4.8 G FAT, 5.9 G CARBOHYDRATES, 15 G PROTEIN

 ERIN SAYS: *"I love all kinds of mushrooms, and substituting shiitake mushrooms in this dish makes it even more fabulous. Plus, shiitake mushrooms can boost your immune system."*

ROCKIN' FACT Spinach is a great source of energy-boosting iron. Make sure to have some form of vitamin C when you eat it to increase the iron's absorption.

Pretty Pomodoro Frittata

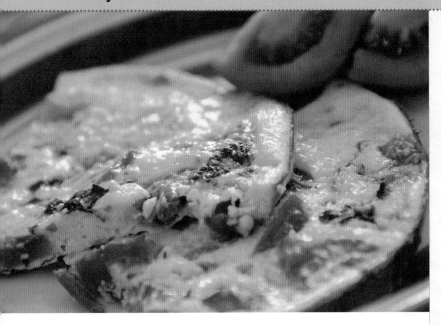

Makes 4 servings ~

3 eggs + 3 egg whites, whisked together

½ cup nonfat milk

3 Roma tomatoes, seeded and chopped

½ cup basil, cut thin

¼ cup fresh parmesan cheese

3 cloves garlic, minced

Directions:

1. Preheat oven to 350°F. Coat a glass pie plate with canola oil cooking spray.
2. Whisk all ingredients together in a large bowl and pour into the pie plate. Place in oven and bake 25 minutes or until eggs are set.
3. Remove and let cool 5 minutes before slicing into wedges.

NUTRIENTS PER SERVING: 121 CALORIES, 6.6 G FAT, 5 G CARBOHYDRATES, 0.7 G FIBER, 9 G PROTEIN

ROCKIN' FACT Adding fresh herbs to any recipe is the key to boosting flavor without having to add salt.

ERIN SAYS: *"I love a recipe that I can eat all week long. Cook once, eat four times. Great for breakfast, lunch, or dinner; hot or cold. Now that's smart planning."*

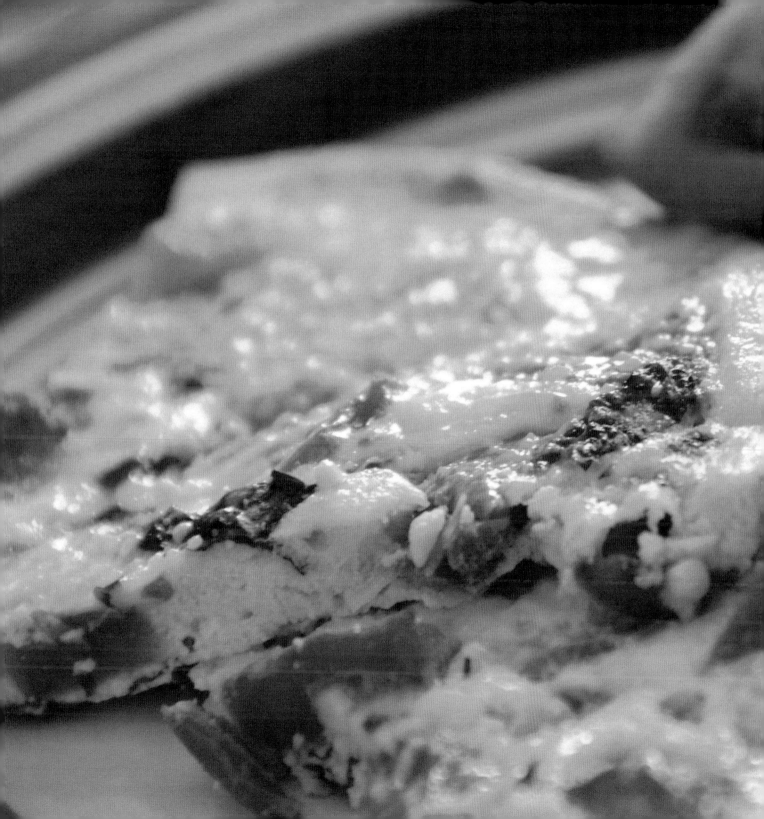

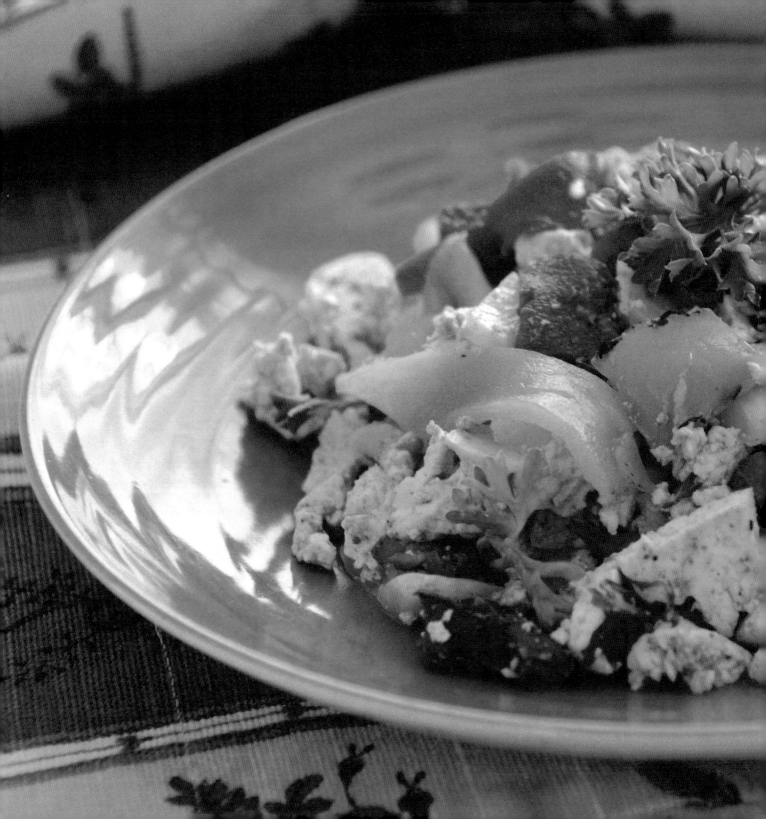

"I'm Doomed to be Heavy Because of My Genes"

"I never can get thin… it drives me crazy! Even at my thinnest I am still big. You know, heavier build, thick waist, wide hips. It's in my genes. I'm just predisposed to being BIG. How can I lose some weight around my belly? Help!"

Yes, it's true. We do come in different sizes and shapes. And if the above quote sounds like we're reading your mind, YOU, my friend, have characteristics of an endomorph. You may have always struggled to lose weight and are genetically prone to storing fat easily. But have no fear. We have the secret to taking that beautiful body of yours and enhancing it to a tighter and sexier you. Yes, you will need to pay more attention to what you eat and how you exercise, but the good news is that it is totally possible to get lean.

A body like yours will do best when it limits (better yet, eliminates) all processed and simple carbohydrates (sweets and white flour products and pasta, white rice, potatoes) as these cause a rapid rise of your blood sugar level which in turn triggers the release of insulin, the fat-storage hormone. Your nutrition plan for losing weight should be focused on plant-based carbs (veggies and fruit, especially berries), lean quality protein (chicken/turkey breast, fish, lean beef, whey protein, egg) and healthy fats, such as omega 3 sources (fish, seafood) and especially virgin coconut oil, which helps to increase your sluggish metabolism. To keep your metabolic rate up, be sure to divide your daily meals into smaller portions so that you have something to eat handy every 2-3 hours.

TIFFANI AND ERIN'S LIFESTYLE TIPS

BE PREPARED! When you're on the go after your workout, make sure to bring an insulated cooler along with you so that you have your post-workout meal ready to go. It can keep cold foods cold or hot foods hot. Then, there's no excuse for skipping a meal or having to stop by a fast-food joint for your food.

CHEW MORE, WEIGH LESS. A study suggests that people who chew their food 40 times vs. the typical 15 times consume 12% fewer calories, which can lead to weight loss. More chewing also affects hormones that control your hunger and fullness, releasing fewer hunger hormones and more fullness hormones. Less hunger + fuller faster = less food consumed.

ORGANIC FOODS. You don't have to buy everything organic. Every year, a list of the "dirty dozen" (most pesticide-laden fruits and vegetables) comes out. These are the foods that should be purchased in the organic form, if possible: apples, peaches, spinach, sweet bell peppers, imported nectarines, cucumbers, potatoes, cherry tomatoes, and hot peppers. For more information, check out the Environmental Working Group's website, http://www.ewg.org/release/apples-top-ewgs-dirty-dozen.

DISTRACTION-FREE DINING. Do you eat while watching TV, talking on the phone, checking emails, or surfing the web? If so, you're not alone. When your mind is fixated on a movie or the latest YouTube video, it's shut off from the cues your body gives you when it's full. Once the TV show is over, you don't feel satisfied because you don't remember what you ate. Power down the electronics and tune into your meal. Listen to the cues your body is giving you. Eat more if you're still hungry and stop when it's full.

Tofu Scrambler

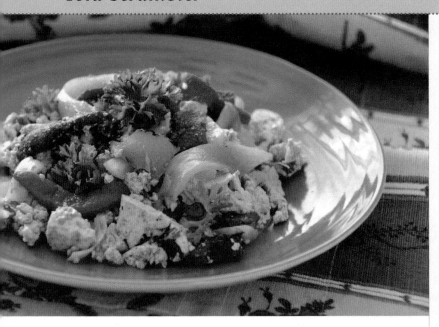

Chapter 6

ROCKIN' FACT Turmeric is known to be anti-inflammatory. It helps with managing pain, boosts brain health, and aids liver detoxification. Most turmeric is found in the spice aisle (bright yellow powder) and can also be found in the fresh produce section in ethnic markets - it looks a lot like it's cousin, ginger.

ERIN SAYS: *"Most people I know are terrified of tofu. In my cooking classes, I've shown how to cook it like eggs, which most people feel comfortable doing. Plus, tofu takes on the flavor of whatever you season it with, so don't be afraid to use lots of herbs and spices."*

Makes 6 servings ~

2 (14-oz.) blocks extra-firm tofu
1 Tbsp. virgin coconut oil
1 small onion, chopped
1 small red bell pepper, finely chopped
½ teaspoon ground cumin
1 ½ teaspoons ground turmeric
1 (15-oz.) can black beans, rinsed, drained
¼ cup coarsely-chopped fresh cilantro
- Kosher salt, freshly ground pepper
- Garnishes: salsa, chopped avocado, sliced scallions, and hot pepper sauce

Directions:

1. Place tofu on a plate lined with several layers of paper towels (to absorb liquid). Using a fork or potato masher, smash tofu.

2. Heat oil in a large skillet over medium-high heat. Add onion and peppers; cook, stirring occasionally, until softened, 3-4 minutes. Stir in cumin; cook until fragrant, about 1 minute. Stir in tofu, then turmeric. Add beans; cook, stirring often, until heated through, 1-2 minutes. Stir in cilantro; season with salt and pepper.

3. Serve with tortillas and garnishes, as desired.

NUTRIENTS PER SERVING: 240 CALORIES, 9.4 G FAT, 17.8 G CARBOHYDRATES, 6.03 G FIBER, 18.14 G PROTEIN

Green Eggs (No, ham. Sorry, SAM I AM!)

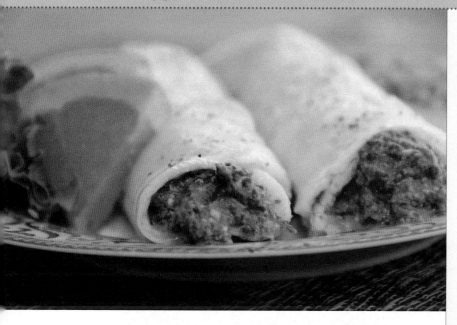

Makes 1 serving ~

4 egg whites

¼ cup cilantro pesto

 (see Extra Rockin' Recipes 88)

Directions:

1. Coat a small nonstick skillet with cooking spray and place over medium high heat until hot. Add the egg whites and let cook 2 minutes. Slide a spatula under the eggs and flip over; cook another 30-60 seconds.

2. Slide onto a plate and place cilantro pesto down the middle of the egg; roll up and eat.

NUTRIENTS PER SERVING: 90 CALORIES, 1 G FAT, 2.9 G CARBOHYDRATES, 1 G FIBER, 16.3 G PROTEIN

ROCKIN' FACT Cilantro is a powerful detoxifying herb, often used to remove heavy metals from the body. It also helps to undo oxidative damage in the body and may even help to control blood sugar.

ERIN SAYS: *"I absolutely love egg whites. Sometimes I eat them twice a day. Plus, I'm a huge fan of cilantro, so I came up with this cilantro-spinach pesto. If you're one of those cilantro-haters, then substitute basil in the recipe."*

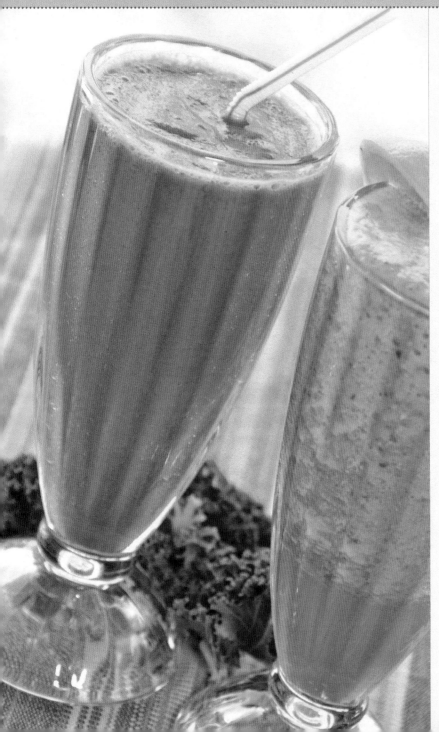

Makes 1 serving ~

2 cups baby spinach

1 cup unsweetened vanilla almond milk

1 banana, frozen and broken into chunks

1 Tbsp. chia seeds

- ice

Directions:

1. Place everything except ice into a blender and blend until smooth. Add the ice cubes, a few at a time, until desired consistency is reached.

NUTRIENTS PER SERVING: 239 CALORIES, 0.6 G FAT, 37 G CARBOHYDRATES, 10.6 G FIBER, 7.3 G PROTEIN

ROCKIN' FACT Almond milk is fortified with calcium and vitamin D

Green Goddess

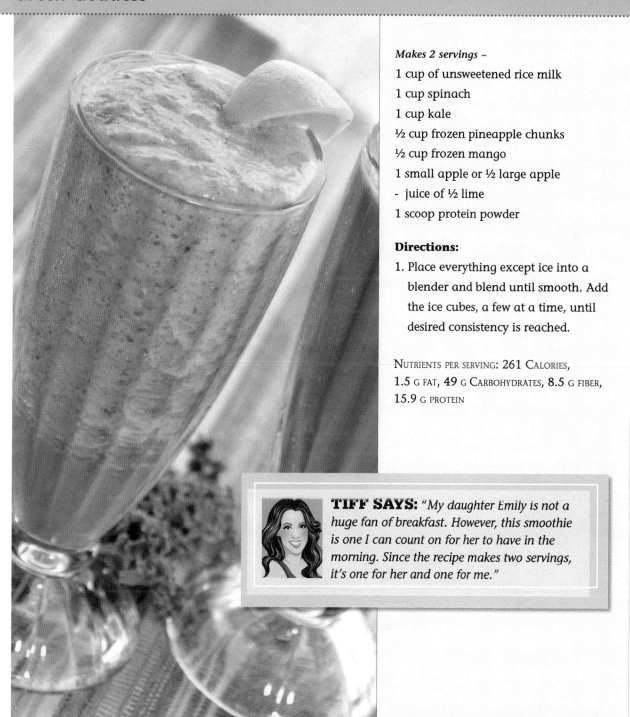

Makes 2 servings ~

1 cup of unsweetened rice milk

1 cup spinach

1 cup kale

½ cup frozen pineapple chunks

½ cup frozen mango

1 small apple or ½ large apple

- juice of ½ lime

1 scoop protein powder

Directions:

1. Place everything except ice into a blender and blend until smooth. Add the ice cubes, a few at a time, until desired consistency is reached.

NUTRIENTS PER SERVING: 261 CALORIES, 1.5 G FAT, 49 G CARBOHYDRATES, 8.5 G FIBER, 15.9 G PROTEIN

TIFF SAYS: *"My daughter Emily is not a huge fan of breakfast. However, this smoothie is one I can count on for her to have in the morning. Since the recipe makes two servings, it's one for her and one for me."*

Tomato, Onion, Green Chile Scrambled Eggs

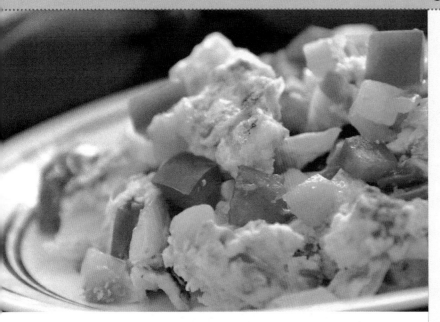

Makes 1 serving ~

1 egg + 3 egg whites, whisked together
1 Roma tomato, chopped and seeded
¼ cup sweet yellow onion, chopped
2 Tbsp. diced green chilies
  (such as Ortega brand)

Directions:

1. Coat a small nonstick skillet with cooking spray and place over medium-high heat until hot. Add the onion, tomatoes, and chilies and cook 2 minutes, until soft.
2. Add the eggs to the pan and let the eggs cook until the bottom is set. Slide a spatula under the eggs and flip over; cook 30-60 seconds. Slide onto a plate and fold in half.

NUTRIENTS PER SERVING: 179 CALORIES, 6.5 G FAT, 13.2G CARBOHYDRATES, 2.2 G FIBER, 18.9 G PROTEIN

TIFF SAYS: *"This is my go-to omelet when I want an easy, healthy, lower-carb breakfast before I hit the gym."*

ROCKIN' FACT The health benefits of tomatoes are boosted by cooking

Nany Sony's LEO – Lox, Eggs, and Onions

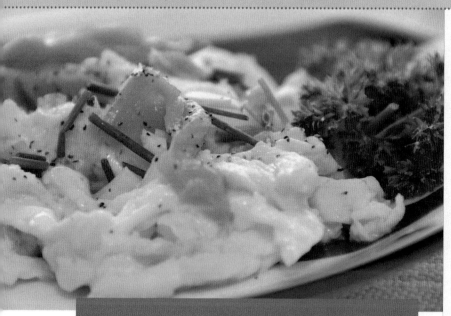

Makes 1 serving ~

1 egg + 2 egg whites

1/4 cup chopped onion

1 oz. smoked salmon, chopped

1 Tbsp. chopped chives

Directions:

1. In a bowl, whisk together egg and egg whites; set aside.

2. Coat a small nonstick skillet with cooking spray and place over medium-high heat until hot. Add the onions and cook about 2 minutes, then add the smoked salmon and cook another 1 minute. Add the eggs to the pan and cook until the bottom sets. Sprinkle the chopped chives on the eggs.

3. Slide a spatula under the eggs and flip over. Cook an additional 30-60 seconds. Slide onto a plate and fold in half.

NUTRIENTS PER SERVING: 166 CALORIES, 6.9 G FAT, 5.3 G CARBOHYDRATES, 0.8 G FIBER, 20.8 G PROTEIN

ROCKIN' FACT Salmon is one of the best sources of anti-inflammatory omega-3 fats. Wild, Alaskan salmon is the cleanest variety of salmon on the market. Steer clear of farm-raised Atlantic salmon - it's much lower in omega-3s and higher in contaminants.

TIFF SAYS: *"This dish reminds me of my grandmother. The first time I had it was when I was a kid and my grandparents would take me out to our local deli for breakfast. In the years before she passed, we would go out to eat at her favorite deli and I'd watch her order it and love every bite!"*

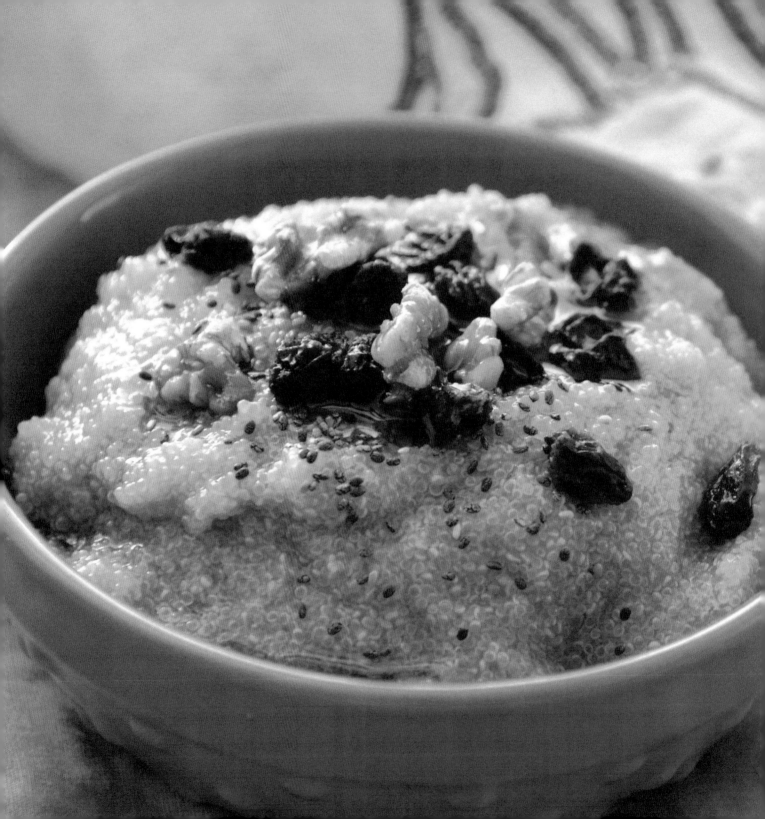

"I Exercise All of the Time . . . I Can Eat What I Want, Right?"

How many times have you thought to yourself, "Hey, I worked out today, I can eat whatever I want!" If you are exercising with the goal of seriously changing your body, this is not a good mindset to have. In fact, it almost guarantees your body will stay exactly as it is regardless of how much you work out. In this case, you're using exercise to stay one step ahead of what are likely poor eating patterns that have become a habit. Your food consumption and exercise programs are not working with each other and are, in fact, in conflict. By far, the biggest complaint we hear from our clients who exercise regularly is that no matter how much they work out, they are not seeing the desired results.

One reason is the widespread belief that to lose weight we must over-exercise while drastically cutting calories or consuming unhealthful diet products. The problem is that when we top off huge calorie-burning workouts with caloric restrictions, we often wind up bingeing or craving high-calorie processed foods loaded with fat and sugar. Once this happens, we've lost the power of conscious choice as our hunger literally takes over our bodies.

By using exercise as a means to either overeat or eat foods that don't properly fuel your body, you rob yourself of the benefits from all of those hours spent at the gym. A healthy pre-workout breakfast provides necessary fuel for those early morning workouts (you will not burn more fat exercising on an empty stomach). A well-balanced post-workout breakfast will refuel your body (so you can go at it again tomorrow) and repair damaged muscle tissue. All-in-all, incorporating a smart, satiating breakfast creates a strong foundation on which you can build for the rest of the day.

EAT APPROXIMATELY 200-400 CALORIES
60 - 120 minutes before you exercise

If you're lucky enough to have one to two hours before you exercise, then you have many more options for the type of meal you can eat to provide you with the fuel you need. The focus of your pre-workout meal should be on slow-digesting complex carbohydrates, which provide you with the fuel that you need, and some lean protein, which stabilizes your blood sugar for longer, keeping you more energized during your entire workout. You'll probably need to eat 200-400 calories, depending on how far out you are from exercising, and the planned intensity of your workout. If it's only an hour until you exercise, then you can aim for the lower end of the calorie spectrum, but if it looks like your workout is two hours away, make sure you consume the extra calories. Think of calories like how many of gallons of gas you put into your car. If you put in a full tank (more calories), you be able to go farther and workout harder.

You're short on time but you know you have to eat something before you exercise. Check out these quick ideas which will fuel your body for a great workout.

Quick-digesting fuel for early morning workout: 15-30 minutes before your workout
Focus on high-glycemic, simple carbohydrates. Low in fat, fiber, and protein.

- 1/3 banana spread with 1/2 Tbsp. almond butter | 83 CALORIES, 4 G FAT, 10 CARBOHYDRATES, 2 G FIBER, 2 G PROTEIN

- 1 rice cake with 1/2 Tbsp. almond butter | 88 CALORIES, 4 G FAT, 10 CARBOHYDRATES, 1 G FIBER, 3 G PROTEIN

- Blend 1/2 scoop whey protein powder, ½ c strawberries with 6 oz. unsweetened almond milk
  94 CALORIES, 3 G FAT, 8 G CARBOHYDRATES, 2 G FIBER, 9 G PROTEIN

- 1/2 piece of fruit + 1 Tbsp. sunflower seeds | 87 CALORIES, 5 G FAT, 9 CARBOHYDRATES, 2 G FIBER, 2 G PROTEIN

Quick-digesting fuel when you have 30-60 minutes before your workout
Aim for 150 calories with complex carbohydrates, protein.

- 1 apple + 1 Tbsp. almond butter | 170 CALORIES, 9 G FAT, 19 CARBOHYDRATES, 4 G FIBER, 4 G PROTEIN

- 1/2 banana + 1 Tbsp. natural peanut butter | 148 CALORIES, 8 G FAT, 17 G CARBOHYDRATES, 3 G FIBER, 5 G PROTEIN

- 1 rice cake + 1 Tbsp. peanut or almond butter + 1 tsp. all-fruit preserves | 148 CALORIES, 7 G FAT, 14 G CARBOHYDRATES, 2 G FIBER, 5 G PROTEIN

- Chia smoothie: The night before, mix together 1 Tbsp. chia seed + 8 oz. almond milk + 1/2 scoop protein powder. Shake well and let sit overnight to thicken. | 165 CALORIES, 7 G FAT, 13 G CARBOHYDRATES, 6 G FIBER, 12 G PROTEIN

- Eggs, oats, 'n jam: Whisk together 2 egg whites. Measure 1/4 cup old-fashioned oats and let soak 5 minutes. Heat a pan and coat with cooking spray. Add egg mixture and scramble until done. Top with 1 Tbsp. all-fruit preserves. | 137 CALORIES, 1 G FAT, 21 G CARBOHYDRATES, 2 G FIBER, 9G PROTEIN

Rockin' Raspberry-Banana Oat Cakes

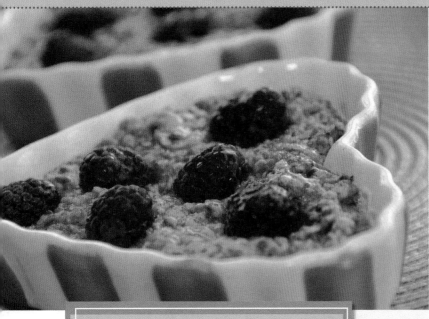

ERIN SAYS: *"I found that the riper the banana, the less sugar, agave, or honey I have to use in the recipe. Plus the banana does double-duty by keeping the cake more moist."*

Makes 4 servings ~

1-¼ cup old-fashioned oats

2 tsp. baking powder

- pinch salt

2 large or 3 small very ripe bananas

1 egg

¼ cup agave nectar

½ tsp. ground cinnamon

1 tsp. vanilla extract

1 Tbsp. chia seed

1 Tbsp. ground flax seed

1 cup berries

Directions:

1. Preheat oven to 350°F.

2. In a medium bowl, place oats, baking powder, and salt. Whisk to combine.

3. In a large mixing bowl, mash the banana with the egg, agave, cinnamon, vanilla extract, chia seed, and flax seed; mix well. Add the dry ingredients to the wet ingredients and gently stir to combine. Fold in the berries.

4. Spray an 8 x 8-inch baking dish with canola oil cooking spray.

5. Pour in the batter and bake in the oven 20-25 minutes or until a toothpick inserted in the center comes out clean or with dry crumbs clinging to it.

6. Remove from oven and let cool 5 minutes before digging in. If you bake them in a baking dish, allow them to cool about 10 minutes before slicing into bars.

7. Best served warm!

NUTRIENTS PER SERVING: **295** CALORIES, **4.6** G FAT, **60** G CARBOHYDRATES, **8.9** G FIBER, **7.1** G PROTEIN

ROCKIN' FACT Bananas are a great source of potassium, an electrolyte that gets lost in your sweat.

Fruit-Filled Crepes – (Apple-Cinnamon, Berry Berry, or Peach-blueberry)

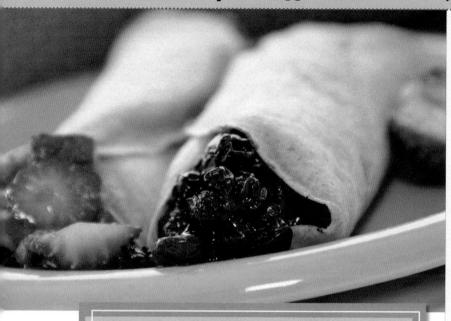

See Extra Rockin' Recipes for fruit filling recipes (pg 86, 87)
Makes 3 servings ~

Whole Wheat Crepes

1 cup whole wheat pastry flour

1 egg, 1 egg white

⅔ cup unsweetened vanilla almond milk

2 Tbsp. raw sugar

1 Tbsp. virgin coconut oil

1 tsp. vanilla

- pinch of salt

¼ cup sparkling water (or club soda)

Directions:

1. Combine all of the ingredients in a medium-mixing bowl. Cover with plastic wrap and place in fridge. Let sit and rest for at least one hour or overnight.

2. Add ½ tsp. coconut oil to a preheated skillet. Swirl skillet to evenly coat with the oil. Add about ⅓ cup batter and swirl the batter in the pan to cover the surface, making a very thin layer of batter; cook about 1 minute or until golden. Flip and cook the other side for 30-45 seconds.

3. Remove from skillet and fill each crepe with ¼ cup fruit compote of choice.

ERIN SAYS: *"Crepe making is really a family affair. Because the cooking of the crepes happens pretty quickly, I have my kids help me out by filling and folding them as soon as they come out of the pan."*

ROCKIN' FACT Sparkling water is the secret ingredient to having the right texture and lacy structure of crepes.

NUTRIENTS PER CREPE (NO FILLING): 126 CALORIES, 3.7 G FAT, 19.2 G CARBOHYDRATES, 2.1 G FIBER, 3 G PROTEIN

1 SERVING = 2 CREPES + ½ CUP COMPOTE FILLING

Bite this Bacon Quesadilla!

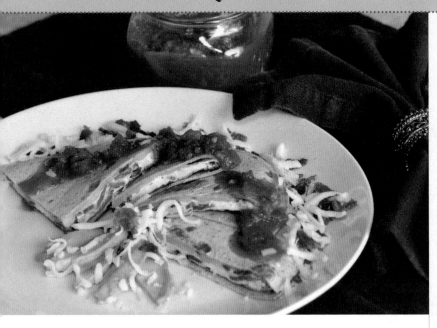

Makes 1 serving ~

1 egg + 2 egg whites, scrambled

1 whole wheat tortilla

1 slice turkey bacon, cooked and crumbled

2 Tbsp. shredded part-skim mozzarella cheese

2 Tbsp. salsa (spicy or mild)

¼ avocado, sliced

Directions:

1. Coat a nonstick pan with cooking spray and place over medium-high heat.
2. Place a whole wheat tortilla in the hot pan and layer the cheese, egg, and crumbled turkey bacon onto one half. Fold the other half over and press down with a spatula. Cook 1 minute and flip; cook another minute.
3. Remove to a plate and top with salsa and avocado slices.

NUTRIENTS PER SERVING: 359 CALORIES, 14.1 G FAT, 267.1G CARBOHYDRATES, 4.5 G FIBER, 31.3 G PROTEIN

TIFF SAYS: *"This is another one of my favorite weekend breakfast recipes. I usually eat this breakfast quesadilla 1 1/2 to 2 hours before a high-intensity workout."*

ROCKIN' FACT Boosting the volume of the egg with two egg whites not only boosts the protein but makes the quesadilla much more hearty.

Nutty & Fruity Amaranth Hot Cereal

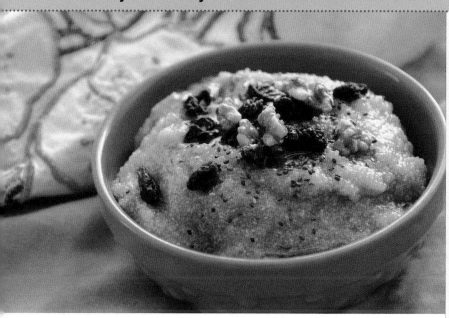

Makes 1 serving ~

⅓ cup amaranth

⅔ cup water

¼ cup rice milk

¼ cup dried cranberries

1 Tbsp. chopped nuts (almonds, walnuts, or pistachios)

1 Tbsp. chia seeds

Directions:

1. Bring the water to a boil in a pot and add the amaranth. Cover and reduce heat to a simmer and cook until the water is absorbed. Stir in the rice milk, cranberries, nuts and chia seeds.

2. Pour into a bowl and serve.

NUTRIENTS PER SERVING: 333 CALORIES, 11 G FAT, 51 G CARBOHYDRATE, 8 G PROTEIN

TIFF SAYS: *"I often add a little almond or vanilla extract to the amaranth while it's cooking or stir in a little orange zest to really give it a bright flavor."*

ROCKIN' FACT Amaranth is not a grain; it's really a seed, which makes it a really balanced food - clean carbs, high in protein, fiber, and omega 3s.

Maple-Blueberry Muffin

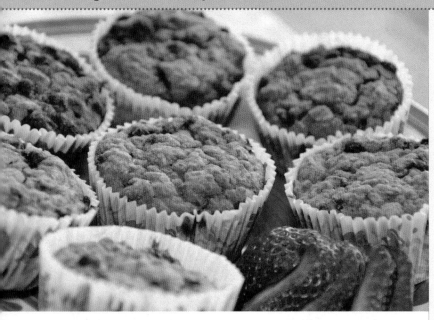

Makes 12 muffins ~

1 ¼ cup whole wheat pastry flour

2 tsp. baking powder

- Pinch salt

1 cup unsweetened applesauce

1 egg

¼ cup pure maple syrup

½ tsp. ground cinnamon

1 tsp. vanilla extract

1 Tbsp. chia seed

1 Tbsp. ground flax seed

1 cup organic blueberries
   (fresh or frozen, thawed)

Directions:

1. Preheat oven to 350°F.

2. In a medium bowl, combine flour, baking powder, and salt. Whisk to combine.

3. In a large mixing bowl, mash the applesauce with the egg, maple syrup, cinnamon, vanilla extract, chia seed, and flax seed; mix well. Add the dry ingredients to the wet ingredients and gently stir to combine. Gently fold in the blueberries. Do not overmix!

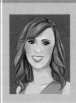

ERIN SAYS: *"My kids love muffins and it's a great snack for after a tough game or practice. Plus, I'm a rock-star mom when I make a few batches for the whole team!"*

4. Spray a muffin tin with canola oil cooking spray. Fill each muffin opening about ⅔ full; place in the oven and bake for 15-18 minutes or until light golden color on top and a toothpick inserted into the middle of a muffin comes out clean or with dry crumbs clinging to it.
5. Remove from oven and let cool 5 minutes in pan; remove and place on baking rack to cool completely.
6. Best served warm!

NUTRIENTS PER 1 MUFFIN: 93 CALORIES, 1.1 G FAT, 18.5 G CARBOHYDRATES, 2.4 G FIBER, 2.2 G PROTEIN

ROCKIN' FACT Blueberries have more antioxidants than any other fruit and really do a body good - they can banish belly fat, boost heart health, reduce risk of cancer, improve bone mass, preserve your vision, and improve your memory.

Chocolate PB Banana Shake

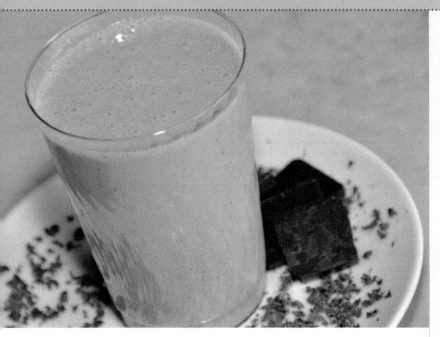

Makes 1 serving ~

1 cup unsweetened vanilla
  almond milk

1 scoop chocolate protein powder

1 banana (frozen)

1 Tbsp. peanut or almond butter

- Ice, if necessary

Directions:

1. Place all ingredients into a blender
   and blend until smooth. Add ice
   for a thicker shake.

NUTRIENTS PER SERVING: 360 CALORIES,
13.4 G FAT, 35.5 G CARBOHYDRATES,
5.6 G FIBER, 29.3 G PROTEIN

TIFF SAYS: *"I know I'm crazy for the flavor combo of chocolate and peanut butter - who isn't? There's a whole industry devoted to it!"*

ROCKIN' FACT One 8-oz. serving of original unsweetened almond milk if fortified with vitamins A and D, are naturally low in fat and contains only 40 calories and 0 grams of sugar.

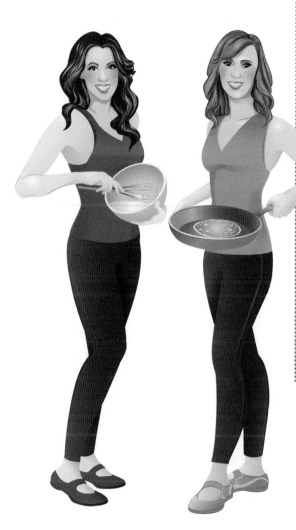

YOUR IDEAL TIMING TO REFUEL
is within 30 – 60 minutes Post-Workout

The post workout meal is probably your most important meal of the day. The purpose of this meal is to refuel, replenish, repair, and rebuild. When you work out, two major things happen: 1) You create micro tears in your muscle fibers which need to be repaired; and 2) you deplete your glycogen stores. When you workout, your primary fuel is glycogen, which is your body's stored form of carbohydrate. Glycogen is like the gas in the fuel tank in your car. When you use it up, you need to fill it back up. Sports nutrition experts have determined that there is a "window" of 30-60 minutes immediately post-workout in which maximal glycogen synthesis occurs. The ideal post-workout meal needs to have both carbohydrates and protein, usually in a 3:1 or 4:1 ratio, for glycogen synthesis. If your workout happens to be more weights than cardio, then try aiming for more of a 2:1 or 1:1 ratio of carbs to protein. The following recipes have been created to maximize glycogen storage and repair damaged muscle tissue.

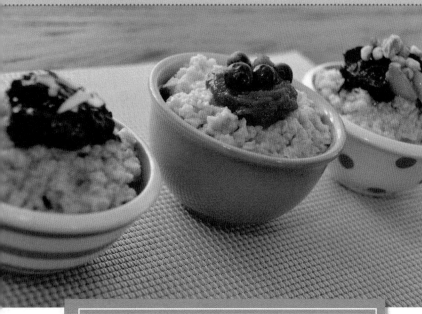

ERIN SAYS: *"I like to cook my oatmeal in milk or soymilk, which really boosts the protein content of this recipe. But be aware that cooking it in the microwave with milk can cause it to overflow, so cook it in an extra large bowl to prevent an oatmeal explosion."*

ROCKIN' FACT Oats have been shown in scientific studies to favorably alter metabolism and improve athletic performance.

Each makes 1 serving ~

½ cup old-fashioned oats (or steel-cut or Irish)

1 Tbsp. chia seeds

1 cup water

½ cup fruit filling (berry compote, blueberry-peach compote, or ¼ cup pumpkin butter) (*see Extra Rockin' Recipes pages 86, 87 and 90*)

Directions:

1. Combine oats, chia seeds, and water in a microwave-safe bowl. Cook on HIGH for 2 minutes. Stir in fruit filling and microwave an additional 30-60 seconds.

2. Stove-top cooking: Combine oats, chia seeds, and water in a saucepan and place on stove over medium-high heat. Stir until oats are cooked, about 5 minutes. Stir in fruit filling and cook an additional 1 minute.

3. Remove from heat and serve.

NUTRIENTS PER SERVING: 275 CALORIES, 5.7 G FAT, 48.2 G CARBOHYDRATES, 9.6 G FIBER, 8.4 G PROTEIN

Pumpkin Pie Shake

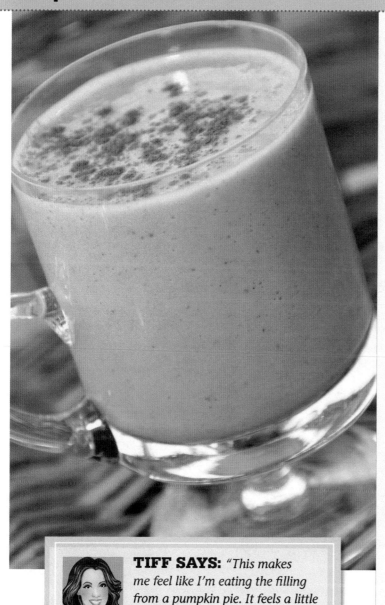

Makes 1 serving ~

1 cup unsweetened vanilla almond
  milk, rice milk, or soy milk (non GMO)
½ cup canned pumpkin
1 scoop vanilla protein powder
½ tsp. cinnamon
¼ tsp. nutmeg
- ice cubes

Directions:

1. Place all ingredients, except ice, into
   a blender and blend until smooth.
2. Add ice cubes, one at a time, and
   continue to blend until shake reaches
   desired consistency.

NUTRIENTS PER SERVING: 170 CALORIES,
0 G FAT, 15 G CARBOHYDRATE, 6 G FIBER,
23 G PROTEIN

ROCKIN' FACT Pumpkin
is a "smart carb" and a great
source of antioxidants and
belly-filling fiber.

TIFF SAYS: *"This makes
me feel like I'm eating the filling
from a pumpkin pie. It feels a little
naughty but it's oh-so-nice for
your body."*

Strawberry Banana Yogurt Parfait

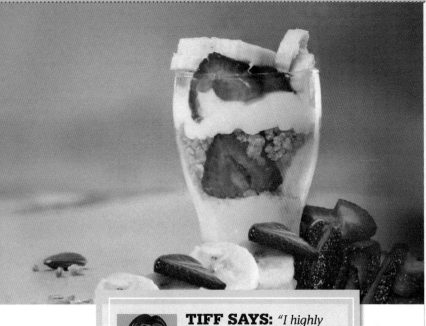

Makes 1 serving ~

1 cup nonfat plain Greek yogurt

- zest of ¼ orange

⅛ tsp. cinnamon

¼ tsp. vanilla extract

1 tsp. honey

½ banana, sliced

½ cup strawberries, sliced

1 Tbsp. chia seeds

2 Tbsp. low-sugar granola

Directions:

1. Stir together yogurt, orange zest, cinnamon, vanilla, and honey.

2. Place half of yogurt in bottom of bowl, top with half of the fruit slices, chia seeds, and granola; repeat with remaining yogurt, fruit, chia seeds, and granola.

NUTRIENTS PER SERVING: 365 CALORIES, 5.46 G FAT, 58.7 G CARBOHYDRATES, 9.7G FIBER, 25.9 G PROTEIN

TIFF SAYS: *"I highly recommend this recipe to my clients for a post workout breakfast when they had a really long or hard workout."*

ROCKIN' FACT Studies show that yogurt eaters have smaller waist sizes than their counterparts (as part of a healthy calorie-controlled eating plan).

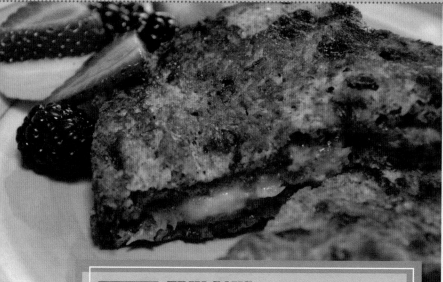

Directions:

1. Coat a nonstick pan with canola oil cooking spray and place over medium-high heat until hot. When hot, add the banana slices; cook 2 minutes per side, or until golden.

2. Spread the almond butter on one of the slices of bread. Place the cooked banana slices on top of the almond butter. Place the second slice of bread on top of the bananas.

3. In a flat-bottomed dish, combine the egg, almond milk, vanilla extract, agave, and cinnamon. Add the sandwich to the mixture and allow to soak for 1 minute on each side.

4. Coat the pan again with cooking spray and place over medium-high heat until hot. Remove the sandwich from the soaking liquid and place in the pan; cook 2-3 minutes, or until golden; flip and cook an additional 2-3 minutes or until golden.

5. Remove from pan and place on cutting board. Slice on diagonal into 2 triangles. Serve.

ERIN SAYS: *"This dish was created by my son Alex when he was 10 years old. He absolutely loves cooked bananas and cinnamon raisin French toast. So we decided to combine them and add a little almond butter for extra protein and healthy fat. Voila! A healthful version of an Elvis Classic."*

ROCKIN' FACT
Researchers have found that diets rich in cinnamon can help reduce the body's negative responses to eating high-fat meals.

Makes 1 serving ~

2 slices Ezekiel cinnamon raisin bread

1 banana, cut into ½-inch rounds

1 Tbsp. almond butter

2 Tbsp. egg beaters or 1 egg

2 Tbsp. unsweetened vanilla almond milk or nonfat milk

½ tsp. vanilla extract

1 tsp. agave nectar

¼ tsp. ground cinnamon

NUTRIENTS PER SERVING: **431** CALORIES, **12** G FAT, **76.2** G CARBOHYDRATES, **8.3** G FIBER, **14.6** G PROTEIN

Chapter 7

Carrot-Ginger Energizing Smoothie

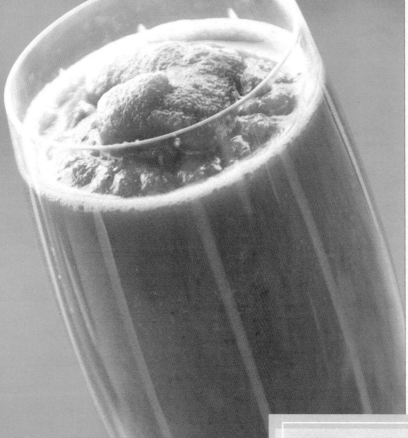

Makes 1 serving ~

1 cup carrot juice

1 apple chopped (your choice whether
to leave on the skin)

1 tsp. fresh grated ginger

1 scoop vanilla protein powder
(whey or vegan)

1 tbs. chia seeds

- ice

Directions:

1. Place all ingredients into a blender
and process until smooth. Add as
much ice as you need to reach the
desired consistency.

NUTRIENTS: 383 CALORIES, 5.0 FAT,
61.1 CARBOHYDRATES, 12.4 FIBER, 21.1 PROTEIN

TIFF SAYS: *"When I feel a cold coming on
I turn to this smoothie because the ginger helps
to get rid of throat and nose congestion. Plus
ginger is full of anti-inflammatory compounds
which really help with muscle soreness."*

ROCKIN' FACT Ginger is
a great digestive aid and can
help out your tummy when
you are feeling nauseous.

Extra Rockin' Recipes

One of our favorite things to do is repurpose recipes so they can be used in a variety of dishes. Spreads like fruit compotes and pumpkin butter make the perfect candidates for doing double and even triple duty! Whip them up and treat yourself all week long to their delicious and unique flavors in different recipes. It's an easy way to liven up your weekly menu and you can even use them as a clean dessert!

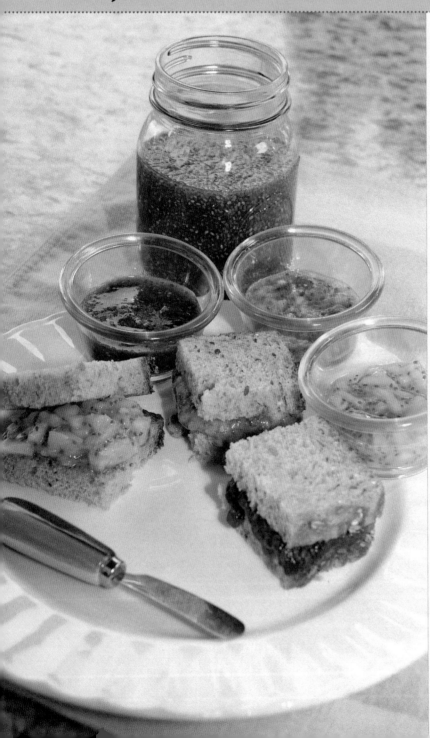

Strawberry Chia Jam

Makes 1 serving (2 Tbsp.) ~
1 cup fresh or frozen (thawed)
    organic strawberries
2 Tbsp. chia seeds
1 tsp. honey

Directions:

1. Place the strawberries in a food
   processor and puree. Remove to a bowl
   and stir in the chia seeds and honey.
   Let sit at least 2 hours before using.

NUTRIENTS PER SERVING: 51 CALORIES,
2.4 G FAT, 7.3 G CARBOHYDRATES, 3.5 G FIBER,
1.3 G PROTEIN

Mango Chia Jam

Makes 1 serving (2 Tbsp.) ~
1 ripe mango or 2 cups frozen mango, thawed
2 Tbsp. chia seeds

Directions:

1. Place mango in a food processor and puree. Remove to a bowl and stir in the chia seeds. Let sit at least 2 hours before using

NUTRIENTS PER SERVING: 33 CALORIES, 1.25 G FAT, 5.0 G CARBOHYDRATES, 1.8 G FIBER, 0.6 G PROTEIN

Banana Chia Jam

Makes 1 serving (2 Tbsp.) ~
1 ripe banana
2 Tbsp. chia seeds
1 tsp. honey or agave syrup

Directions:

1. Place banana in food processor and puree. Remove to a bowl and stir in chia seeds and honey or agave. Let sit at least 2 hours before serving.

NUTRIENTS PER SERVING: 65 CALORIES, 2.35 G FAT, 11.17 G CARBOHYDRATES, 3.53 G FIBER, 1.3 G PROTEIN (FOR ½ CUP YIELD)

Berry Compote

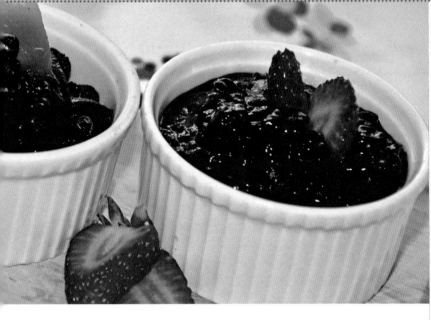

Makes 8 servings ~

2 cups fresh or frozen mixed organic
   berries (strawberries, raspberries,
   blueberries, blackberries)
1 tsp. lemon zest
- zest of ½ orange
1 Tbsp. agave or honey

Directions:

1. Place all ingredients in a pan on
   the stove over medium heat. Cook
   until berries release their juices,
   about 5 minutes.
2. Mix ½ Tbsp. cornstarch into 1 Tbsp.
   cold water until dissolved.
3. Pour into the berry mixture and stir
   until thickened. Remove from heat
   and cool 5 minutes.

NUTRIENTS PER 2 TABLESPOONS: 25 CALORIES,
0.13 G FAT, 6.38 G CARBOHYDRATES,
1.25 G FIBER, 0.25 G PROTEIN

Blueberry Peach Compote

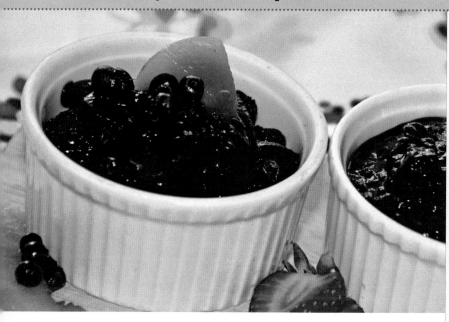

Makes 8 servings ~

1 cup fresh or frozen organic blueberries

1 cup fresh or frozen organic peaches

½ tsp. cinnamon

Directions:

1. Place all ingredients into a saucepan over medium-high heat. Cook until fruit starts to release its juices, then lower heat to Low and simmer until thickened, about 15 minutes

NUTRIENTS PER 2 TABLESPOONS: 22 CALORIES, 0.1 G FAT, 4.5 G CARBOHYDRATES, 1 G FIBER, 0.3 G PROTEIN (1 CUP YIELD)

Cilantro Pesto

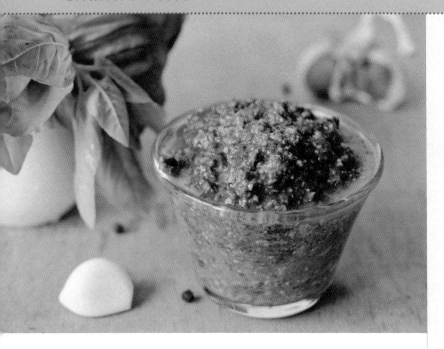

Makes 1 serving (1/4 c)

1 10-oz. bag frozen spinach, thawed
   and pressed against a fine-mesh
   strainer to remove as much water
   as possible

1 cup organic cilantro

- zest of 1 lemon (organic)

- juice of 1 lemon

½ cup nonfat plain Greek yogurt

2 Tbsp. parmesan cheese

Directions:

1. Place in a food processor and puree.
   Remove to a bowl.

NUTRIENTS PER SERVING: 22 CALORIES,
0.7 G FAT, 1.9 G CARBOHYDRATES, 1 G FIBER,
1.9 G PROTEIN

Yogurt Cheese

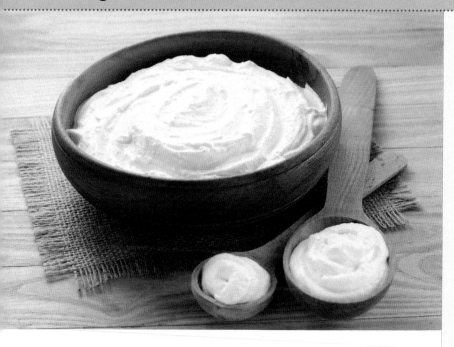

- 32-oz. plain nonfat yogurt (make sure it is a brand with NO gelatin)
- cheesecloth
- strainer & bowl

Directions:

1. Place 8 layers of cheesecloth in the strainer and place strainer over a bowl. Pour the yogurt into the cheesecloth and place bowl in the refrigerator. Let drain 12 - 24 hours, depending on the consistency desired.

NUTRIENTS PER 1 TBSP.: 23 CALORIES, 0 G FAT, 3.2 G CARBOHYDRATES, 0 G FIBER, 2.3 G PROTEIN

Pumpkin Butter

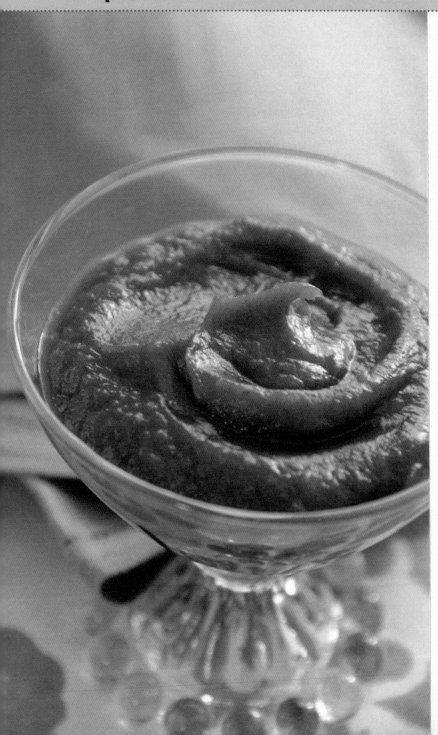

Makes approx. 2 cups

15-oz. can pumpkin puree

½ cup honey

1 Tbsp. pure maple syrup

½ tsp. pure vanilla extract

1 tsp. cinnamon

- zest of ¼ orange

- pinch of salt

Directions:

1. Combine all ingredients in a small saucepan over medium-low heat, mixing until well combined.
2. Stir constantly, cook for about 15 minutes, or until thickened.
3. Remove the pan from heat, and transfer your pumpkin butter to a small bowl or jar. Let cool completely before covering and refrigerating.

NUTRIENTS PER 2 TBSP.: 43 CALORIES, 0 G FAT, 11.7 G CARBOHYDRATES, 1.3 G FIBER, 0.5 G PROTEIN

Your No Excuses Shopping List: What to Stock Up On

Your No Excuses Shopping List: What to Stock Up On

NOTE: In some instances, we provide brand names to make it easier for you to find a good product. We are not sponsored by any of these brands, and if you find a worthy alternative you prefer, more power to you!

Pantry
- Canned pumpkin
- Evaporated skim milk
- Black beans
- Salsa verde
- Canned diced green chilies
- Almond butter *(preferably raw, refrigerate after opening)*
- Natural peanut butter
- Organic marinara sauce
- Hot sauce
- All-fruit preserves
- Raw agave nectar
- Date sugar
- Raw honey
- Pure maple syrup
- Raw walnut pieces *(best to store in refrigerator)*
- Raw almonds *(best to store in refrigerator)*
- Raw sunflower seeds *(best to store in refrigerator)*
- Chia seeds *(best to store in refrigerator)*
- Flax seeds, ground *(best to store in refrigerator)*
- Hemp hearts *(best to store in refrigerator)*
- Oats *(steel cut and old-fashioned)*
- Healthy granola *(Nature's Path Organic Hemp Plus, Kashi Go Lean Crunch)*
- Whole wheat tortillas
- Sprouted grain tortillas
- Corn tortillas
- Sprouted grain bread *(Ezekiel)*
- Whole wheat english muffin
- Amaranth *(best to store in refrigerator)*
- Virgin coconut oil
- Extra, unrefined virgin olive oil
- Canola oil
- Grape seed oil
- Whey protein powder *(chocolate, vanilla)*
- Cocoa powder
- Whole wheat pastry flour
- Baking powder
- Baking soda
- Mini semi-sweet chocolate chips
- Raisins
- Brown rice cakes
- Sparkling water *(plain)*

Spices
- Cinnamon
- Nutmeg
- Pure vanilla extract
- Smoked paprika
- Ground cumin
- Turmeric
- Sea salt
- Black pepper

Refrigerator
- Unsweetened vanilla almond milk
- Rice milk
- 1% or nonfat cottage cheese
- Nonfat plain greek yogurt
- Nonfat plain yogurt
- Eggs
- Egg whites
- Fresh salsa
- Non-gmo organic tofu *(extra firm, silken)*
- Smoked salmon or lox
- Orange juice
- Tart cherry juice
- Parmesan cheese
- Oranges
- Avocado
- Organic baby spinach
- Organic kale
- Guacamole

- Organic cilantro
- Onions
- Bell peppers
- Basil
- Lemon
- Lime
- Green onion
- Chives
- Part-skim mozzarella cheese *(sliced or shredded)*
- Chicken-apple sausage *(Applegate breakfast links or Trader Joe's brand)*
- Turkey bacon *(Applegate or any other nitrate-free brand)*

Freezer
- Organic strawberries
- Mango chunks
- Organic chopped spinach
- Skinless, boneless chicken breast
- Chicken or turkey breakfast sausage links *(Applegate or Trader Joe's)*

Produce *(doesn't have to be refrigerated)*
- Organic apples
- Organic berries
- Mushrooms
- Roma tomatoes
- Bananas
- Garlic

Index of Recipes

About the Authors

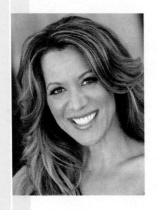

Tiffani Bachus is a Registered Dietitian Nutritionist (RDN), former Fitness America Champion, professional fitness competitor and fitness and nutrition expert dedicated to promoting wellness and inspiring clients to live a healthy balanced lifestyle.

Tiffani is regularly featured on Arizona's 3 TV Good Morning Arizona offering fitness and nutrition tips to viewers. She's been featured as a monthly columnist for the nationally-syndicated Oxygen Magazine, writing the "Easy Does It" column and co-wrote the "Ask the Dietitian" column for Clean Eating Magazine. In addition, Tiffani has sat on the Health Advisory Boards for Clean Eating Magazine.

Tiffani has been featured in, and graced the covers, of numerous fitness magazines including Oxygen Magazine, Scottsdale Health Magazine, Max Sports and Fitness, Fitness Plus Magazine, Natural Muscle, Nutricula Magazine and AZ Living Magazine. She also hosts the annual Arizona show, which features elite fitness competitors from around the country.

In Tiffani's spare time, she can be found teaching dance and fitness classes, practicing yoga and spending time with her husband and three kids.

Tiffani received her B.S. in Nutrition from California State University of Northridge.

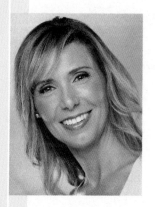

Erin Macdonald, RDN, is a nutrition, fitness, and wellness coach practicing and preaching the nourishment of mind, body, and spirit. She specializes in weight management, sports, cardiovascular, wellness, pregnancy, infant and child nutrition, and food allergy and sensitivity testing.

Erin is a founding member of the Weight Management Dietetic Practice Group, as well as a member of the Academy of Nutrition and Dietetics, Sports, Cardiovascular and Wellness Nutrition (SCAN), Dietitians in Integrative and Functional Medicine (DIFM), and Nutrition Entrepreneurs (NE).

Erin has written regularly for Clean Eating Magazine and Oxygen Magazine, and she is a contributor to Nutricula Magazine - The Science of Longevity. She also has been quoted in numerous magazines and online articles, including Shape.com and Mint.com.

Erin has appeared on radio, television, and DVDs and has presented many lectures focusing on weight management, heart-healthy cooking, sports nutrition, blood sugar health, and pediatric nutrition. Away from work, this native Los Angelino enjoys spending time with her husband and four sons, running, hiking, teaching cooking classes, and having fun.

Erin completed her post-baccalaureate in nutrition sciences from California State University, Los Angeles and received a BA in psychology from UCLA.

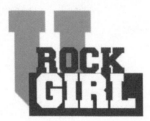

Tiffani Bachus and Erin Macdonald have partnered to co-found U ROCK GIRL, a website dedicated to promoting wellness and a healthy, balanced lifestyle. Their goal is to provide women with tips, recipes and articles aimed at helping them live a healthy lifestyle through proper nutrition, training and wellness. Visit their website at www.urockgirl.com and twitter @urockgirl.

Editor
Joe Bardin
Copy Editor
Karen Kinnison
Front and
Back Cover Photographer
James Patrick
Food Photographer
Alison Plotnik
Food Stylist
Diana Draper
Erin Becker
Graphic Designer
Claudia Gimenez
Illustrator
Greta Schimmel

Printed By
Create Space
Printed in USA

1st Edition January 2014

ISBN: 978-0-9913063-0-5

Visit the U Rock Girl website at
www.urockgirl.com
Twitter
@urockgirl
Facebook
www.facebook.com/URockGirl.URG
Instagram
@u_rock_girl
Email
contactus@urockgirl.com

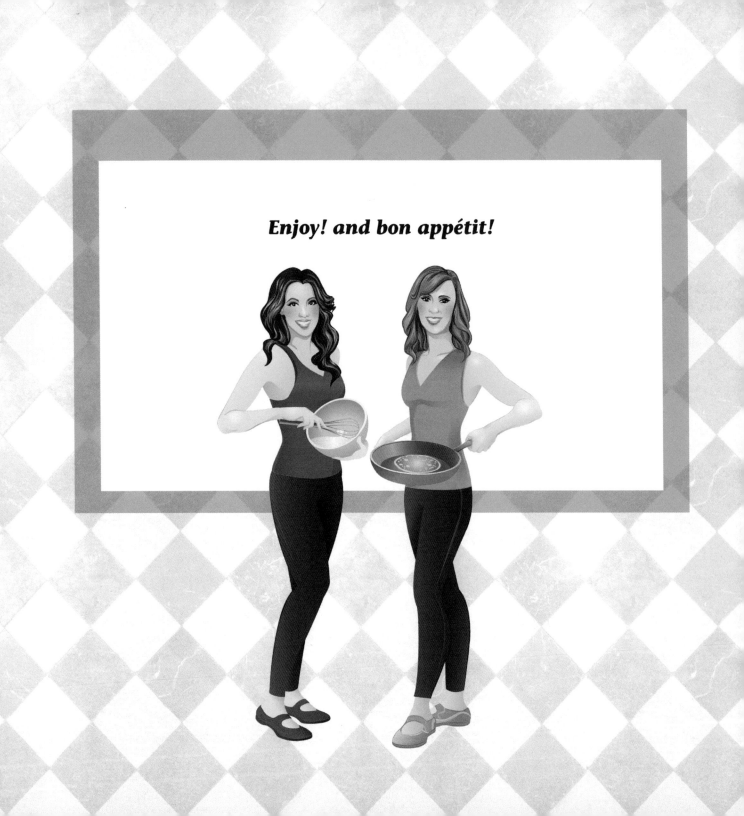

Enjoy! and bon appétit!

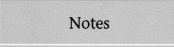

Notes

Notes

Made in the USA
Lexington, KY
17 December 2015